"Dancing from age 11 to 40, I recognized its physical benefits – stronger bones, and cardiovascular health. Dr. Baudino's book revealed how dance and movement have profound mental, emotional, and social benefits, shaping not just a healthy but a happy child."

Nigel Lythgoe, *OBE, PhD*

"This book by Dr. Lori Baudino is a testament to the transformative power of dance movement therapy in promoting psychological and physical health. Providing copious concrete examples in various contexts for a wide variety of neurodevelopmental, behavioral, and psychological issues, Dr. Baudino skillfully navigates the complexities of therapy. Emphasizing the importance of embodied, enactive forms of psychotherapy and expertise in reading what the body is trying to convey, she showcases how dance movement therapy can offer a non-threatening space for children to express themselves."

Dr. Adele Diamond, *PhD,*
FRSC, FAFA, FAPS, FSEP, Sc.D (honoris causa),
D.Phil. (honoris causa)

T0384959

Moving Moments in Childhood

Moving Moments in Childhood provides a roadmap to truly understanding and embodying mental and physical health for children through the lens of dance/movement therapy.

This book explores fifty real therapeutic stories focusing on anxiety, pain, neurodivergence (including the diagnosis of autism spectrum disorder) and learning differences, sibling dynamics, parenting challenges, and chronic illness in childhood. These individualized stories delve into the benefits of supporting the mind/body connection using dance/movement therapy, and each chapter includes diagnostic insights and hands-on strategies to use in therapy sessions, in schools, and at home. The book also includes research on etiology, diagnosis, therapeutic theory, and treatment methodology.

Moving Moments in Childhood highlights the transformative potential of therapeutic movement for a child's mental, physical, social, and psychological health and is an indispensable guide for mental health professionals, educators, and their clients.

Lori Baudino, PsyD, BC-DMT, has been a practicing clinician for over twenty years. Her work fuses integrative health into private practice, hospital care, parent education, and academic development.

DMT with Infants, Children, Teens, and Families

Series Editor: Suzi Tortora, Ed.D, BC-DMT, LCAT a board-certified dance/movement therapist and specialist in the field of infancy mental health and development, has a private dance/movement psychotherapy practice in New York City and Cold Spring, New York.

DMT with Infants, Children, Teens, and Families provides a detailed overview of all the applications of dance/movement therapy nationally and internationally, from its ancient roots in tribal healing rituals to its current uses in medical settings, schools, and private practice to support families and their children, including those with medical illness, generalized anxiety disorders, sensory processing disorders, autism spectrum disorders, eating disorders, trauma, multigenerational trauma, identity issues, and work with immigrants, refugees, people of color and underserviced populations.

The international authors contributing chapters to this series include early innovators, established leaders and young professionals bringing new perspectives to working with children and families. These diverse voices build a discussion about the use of dance to heal children using a multi-cultural lens that is sensitive and inclusive, with full awareness of the underlying influences power, privilege, and oppression have on servicing these populations. Each book includes theoretical/methodological and empirical chapters with many vignettes and case studies illustrating DMT in action in addition to discussing the most prominent innovators in the field both historically and currently.

Dance/Movement Therapy for Infants and Young Children with Medical Illness

Treating Somatic and Psychic Distress
Suzi Tortora and Miri Keren

Moving Moments in Childhood

A Dance/Movement Therapy Lens for Supporting the Whole Child
Lori Baudino with Rachael Singer

For more information about this series, please visit www.routledge.com/ DMT-with-Infants-Children-Teens-and-Families/book-series/DMTI

Moving Moments in Childhood

A Dance/Movement Therapy Lens for
Supporting the Whole Child

Lori Baudino with Rachael Singer

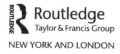
Routledge
Taylor & Francis Group

NEW YORK AND LONDON

Designed cover image & figure images by: Carlos Nietto III

First published 2025
by Routledge
605 Third Avenue, New York, NY 10158

and by Routledge
4 Park Square, Milton Park, Abingdon, Oxon, OX14 4RN

Routledge is an imprint of the Taylor & Francis Group, an informa business

ISBN: 978-1-032-42613-6 (hbk)
ISBN: 978-1-032-42612-9 (pbk)
ISBN: 978-1-003-36349-1 (ebk)

DOI: 10.4324/9781003363491

Typeset in Garamond
by Apex CoVantage, LLC

In loving memory of all the beautiful children who have come into my life and taught me the real meaning of presence, creativity, playfulness, and love. I value each of my interactions, and I am honored and thankful to your caregivers for choosing me to join your family dance.

To my mother for instilling my life with creativity, and to my childhood school/teachers for accepting my mind and my whole self.

To my husband, my daughter, Lyla (and her adorable bunny Jade), and my son, Aiden, for your patience and trust in my parenting.

Contents

Foreword

"Our minds are both embodied and relational and our wellbeing depends upon how we move through physical and social space. Lori Baudino has created a masterful journey for clinicians to explore the art and science of dance/movement therapy in powerful and illuminating detail. In this wonderful compendium of clinical wisdom and practical skills you will find wonderful examples of children and their parents that illustrate how to apply her creative principles of healing with the body in mind. This is a book to guide every child therapist, no matter their background, toward a more holistic and effective approach to supporting development in a healthy direction. Bravo!"

Daniel J. Siegel, M.D.
New York Times Bestselling Author
The Developing Mind; *IntraConnected*; *Mindsight*;
Brainstorm; and *Aware*.
Co-author, *Parenting from the Inside Out*;
The Whole Brain Child and *The Power of Showing Up*
Executive Director, Mindsight Institute
Clinical Professor, UCLA School of Medicine

Preface

Invitation – What If Healing Could Look Like This . . .

This book is a compilation of many "moving moments." The pages you'll read here include answers to the varied questions I have been asked over the years as a practicing psychologist and dance/movement therapist. What does dance/movement therapy actually look like in a therapeutic session? Is this modality really beneficial for connection and health? Is it psychology? How does movement and using the body make a difference for my children?

It is because of my understanding of the mind/body connection that I feel I have made such instrumental connections with the children and families I have met and had the pleasure to support. I believe that the transformative nature of understanding and working with the whole child (mind, body, and spirit) makes for the most growth potential and communication. My desire is to share a year's worth of moments using my embodied attunement with children (my comprehensive dance/movement therapy lens), with hopes of inspiring professionals and families across many fields to seek out and learn how to incorporate the body and movement into our thoughts, interactions, health, and academic models.

These stories are based on real moments, but all names, ages, and identifying information have been changed to ensure confidentiality and safety for all individuals involved. The events are a composite of related scenarios used to illustrate the work and foster understanding of the benefits of supporting children through a mind/body connection. I'm honored to have this opportunity to share and connect with you about healing.

This book identifies the vast range of psychological, cognitive, physical, and social challenges and triumphs of children within the context of the therapeutic dynamic. The vignettes focus on the most prominent cases and clinical experiences. While the book addresses identity, cultural, and individual differences, depending on the sessions, it does not provide a deep dive or a specific expertise regarding race, gender, or identity. Moreover, the emphasis is placed on the therapeutic healing and transformations indicative of movement-based therapeutic interventions for all children.

Throughout this book you will read the words dance/movement with the slash between the words. My intention is (1) to bring attention and support to the field of dance/movement therapy as well as (2) to acknowledge that dance and movement are interchangeable – one and the same. When we move with breath, heartbeat, talking, relating, or larger jumping twirls – we are dancing! Thus, I invite you to replace any fears or preconceived notions of dancing to become an advocate for the true dance of our moving moments.

Additionally, for the dance/movement therapy community, I wanted to thoughtfully honor the discussions and sensitivity around some of the original contributors in our field and your right to discern which theories you continue to use. For my work, I am not following a particular dance/movement therapists' premise, behaviors, or thoughts. Rather I utilize the words around movement to help understand and share how to look at the body. Primarily, I have specifically chosen to use movement terms to understand the emotional and psychological needs from a whole child perspective. I appreciate your attention and collaboration!

Acknowledgment

Special thanks to the Andréa Rizzo Foundation for the chance to provide dance/movement therapy to children with cancer and special needs, a gift that is truly instrumental in making a difference in their lives. My endless appreciation for providing the opportunities to share my passion for dance/ movement therapy with hospitals and children across the country. Lastly, I would like to acknowledge and share my appreciation for Routledge, Suzi Tortora, and Rachael Singer, as this book would not have been possible without your support, and for that, I am immensely grateful.

Let's keep dancing: learn, donate, share – Dreasdream.org.

Introduction

This book introduces Dr. Baudino's aims to collaborate and share the importance of dance/movement therapy for supporting the whole child in clinical work, further expressing the rationale for inviting practitioners, providers, educators, and parents into the lens of embodied healing during this time and onward.

In this book, the author(s)

- Depicts therapeutic vignettes to bring the mental health provider into the therapeutic process of dance/movement therapy, using movement to further one's psychological, mental, physical, emotional, and social integration.
- Offers embodied methodology for neurotypical/neurodiverse populations, including social relationships, individual differences, sibling/family dynamics, and critical child development.
- Provides tangible methods and a framework that reaches across children, gender, class, social economics, race, religion, and abilities.

How to Use This Book

This book invites the reader to step into the therapeutic environment and experience the details of embodied therapeutic healing. By first reading the vignettes, the reader embraces the language, movement, and outcomes within each clinical session and how these pertain to the area of child development. Additional theory and educational research support the framework and applications described.

Why Moving Moments? A Note From the Author

When I was a child, I tap-danced my book report of John Steinbeck's *The Pearl*. Before turning ten, I played basketball to count my math facts and acted out my history lessons. I always knew I would support children – and

DOI: 10.4324/9781003363491-1

that movement was a way to bring meaning to learning and connection to all my relationships.

Forty years later, my vision for integrative health and learning has become more of a reality. Quantum physics, energy healers, doctors, and educators are turning toward mindfulness, movement, exercise, and mental health. Finally, the fluff of dance and movement is the *stuff* of whole child care. Since we know illness, disease, and life success/challenges occur within and between bodies and are expressed through movement, what better way to support health than to start by acknowledging the body as a way to transform challenges and express emotions? The therapy helps one gain control and release discomfort, communicate more effectively, and integrate mind and body. The modality is an adjunct to medical treatment and offers effective tools and awareness for psychological support.

In my clinical work, there are countless hours of interventions with children in which I have looked at the parallel processes of emotional and psychological needs as expressed in the body. The more integrated the medical, academic, and parenting worlds become, the more healthy, connected, and brilliant our children will be. I started writing a moving moments blog because people asked me how dance and movement had anything to do with psychology and mental health. Was I teaching ballet to medically fragile children? Could I help a three-year-old, five-year-old, or ten-year-old manage emotions in therapy?

When you observe my work and experience the awareness of a child's movements, the observations lead to insight, understanding, acceptance, and connection. I started my private practice over twenty years ago; I supervised students, presented at conferences, and created the Collaborative Health Summit (www.drloribaudino.com/summit). Each aspect of my professional development has focused on advocating for mind/body connection for overall health and the use of dance/movement therapy as an integrative and whole child approach to health. Identifying the whole child for me means looking at a child's development by understanding all aspects of that child; learning birth history, sensory processing, movement profile, developmental milestones, visual system, auditory system, oral/motor development, breathing style, nutritional patterns, sleep patterns, toileting history, educational/learning styles, and much more. I ask questions of parents and children to best understand the foundation of what variables play into the child's individual makeup and further where we can support as a team to value and honor the child's experiences, and connections. I see myself as a crusader with a mission to collaborate across disciplines, promoting health through movement, play, and connection. This further supports the wholeness and embodied practices in a field that is over fifty years old: dance/movement therapy.

I believe that mental health and emotional therapy must be celebrated and acknowledged in every home. Every educator and provider needs to learn about the body and movement for education and growth. Moreover, multiple modalities and professional fields working together are more robust and effective than when they are apart. In science, we say integration is differentiated parts that link together; the art and lens of movement allow the child to connect to each movement choice, each body response, to then attach and bring awareness to the body's needs. Ultimately, fostering mental understanding and thus integration (health) occurs. Movement is our innate way of communicating and can reach all people across age range, ethnicity, social-economic class, ability, and gift. *Moving Moments in Childhood: A Dance/Movement Therapy Lens for Supporting the Whole Child* aims to do just that.

Statement of Aims

The pandemic has made mental health and therapeutic intervention necessary now more than ever. Dance/movement therapy can enhance the therapeutic space by using a lens that focuses on the body and movement. Mental health providers and educators can incorporate movement and the integration of mind and body within their practice. The modality of dance/movement therapy forges the way for integrative practices and a whole child focused approach to cognitive, physical, social, and emotional health.

Popular books, like *The Whole-Brain Child* by Dr. Daniel Siegel or *The Conscious Parent* by Dr. Shefali Tsabary, help support parents in becoming their best selves and offer knowledge-based teachings for parent and child development. These books emphasize a top-down approach (the mentalization of emotions) (Siegel & Payne Bryson, 2011; Tsabary, 2010). In this book, the bottom-up approach, identified through dance/movement therapy, highlights how emotions are felt in the body and expressed through movement. This book also encourages providers and educators to be physically in tune with children and to foster the mental preparation for full emotional connection within adult/child relationships. And this book further highlights the relationship between motoric expression and psychological/emotional health.

Moving Moments provides emotionally insightful vignettes to capture the parallels of emotional/mental health and movement expression. The experientials allow for the hands-on application of psychology's most prevalent topics and needs. The book's three tiers – vignettes, therapeutic lens, and experiential activities – will be integral to the intervention process for clinicians and care providers.

References

Siegel, D. J., & Payne Bryson, T. (2011). *The whole-brain child – 12 revolutionary strategies to nurture your child's developing mind.* Bantam Books.

Tsabary, S. (2010). *The conscious parent: Transforming ourselves, empowering our children.* Namaste Pub.

Chapter 1

Critical Areas in Children – Anxiety, Pain, and Neurodivergence

Introduction

As we have been living through the COVID-19 pandemic, which started in early 2020, parents and providers have, more than ever, been observing the manifestation of their own anxieties, pain, and fears while aiming to model a sense of control and consistency for children. This pandemic amplified our health needs and catapulted an awareness of the overwhelming crisis in childhood mental health. When we look at the whole child, when we address the body in a space of connection and communication, support is optimal. Although the current state of the world situation merits anxiety and fear, children may thrive and show their resilience when the body and the brain are met with organization, regulation, and integration. When we view a child's behaviors as movement, we are saying that all of their actions, both physical and verbal, are ways that they are expressing themselves and adapting to their environment. For example, a child who runs away from a dog is moving away from a threat. A child who hugs their parent is moving toward a pleasurable experience. Children's behaviors serve a specific function in the child's life. By understanding the purpose of a child's behaviors, and accepting these actions as movement expressions, we can better understand the child themselves and how to make meaningful connections.

Dance/movement therapy is a powerful modality that can be used to help children with a variety of needs, including those of anxiety, pain, and neurodiversity. As you read the following vignettes, I invite you to explore how this approach can be integrated into your practice to support children's emotional, physical, and social development.

Focus

In each vignette, I aim to highlight the movement patterning, sensory similarities, clinical response, and overall intention of the session. I will also discuss how dance/movement therapy can help us move past diagnosis

DOI: 10.4324/9781003363491-2

and into the fundamental needs of the child. Finally, I will share how this approach can be used to model radical love, attunement, and connection between the therapist, child, and parent. I hope that these vignettes will provide you with a deeper understanding of how dance/movement therapy can be used to help children thrive.

Vignette I: Boiling Beans

"I'm in so much pain I can't do anything."

– Susie, age 15

When I entered the hospital room, Susie was lying in her bed with her fists clenched. She held her body in a tight, straight line. I asked her if we could spend some time participating in dance/movement therapy. She agreed.

We started by thinking about where in her body she felt pain and what it might look like. She described her pain as a "red-brown color, the shape of a bean" located "in her stomach area." I asked if we could gradually start shifting from side to side in a horizontal rocking motion. She moved and described how she had seen this color and shape before, as she recalled how her mom had often cooked beans. Apparently, her mother would spend hours in the kitchen soaking the beans, waiting the whole morning until the beans were ready to be put in a pot to boil.

Susie told me about missing her mom during these hours, but more about how frustrating it was to wait for the beans to cook. Her body stiffened as she expressed her thoughts on frustration and waiting. I asked, "Is this feeling of frustration and waiting familiar in your current daily life?" She explained, as she started to rock more quickly, that waiting was a familiar feeling while she endured her body pains. She could not let it go, nor figure out what the problem was, but she always had the pain.

We continued to rock side to side and discussed how the beans, just like her body before finding relief, would start out stiff and tight before they were soaked. Then I told her to start moving in other directions. In other words, I wanted her to move like beans in an actively boiling pot. This would allow her to lean into and accept her pain, which would then help release it.

Susie undulated from side to side, forward and back, up and down. As this movement increased, we discussed how the water would move as it boiled. She expanded her movement and breathing as she continued to talk with me. "As I am moving," Susie told me, "I feel a softening happening in my body." Eventually, we increased the speed until she felt like her body was completely relaxed and all of her limbs felt soft and fluid. She slowed her body down, took a deep breath – in through her nose, out through her mouth – and finally managed to be still. She said she felt like she didn't have to wait anymore. The pain had disappeared.

At this point, Susie laughed and exclaimed, "I think the beans would be ready to eat!" We laughed together as I had her think about her body, checking her feet, ankles, legs, hips, stomach, back, hands, arms, neck, face, and head to see whether she still had any pain. I then noted that, by making a connection to her pain and allowing her body to move, she appeared to have taken control over her body. In this way, helping her verbally express a change in pain was a wonderful moment.

Vignette 1 Intervention: Boiling Beans

Activity Prompt: Incorporate the following questions to the child within the one-on-one sessions: Where do you feel pain (a change in sensation, a focus point that calls your attention) in your body? Does it have a color, temperature, and shape? Does this area or felt sense move (pulsate, roll, tighten, throb, vibrate)? Does the felt sense remind you of anything in your life? Have you seen this imagery or feeling before?

Provider Note: *Slow down each question for embodied exploration and accurate witnessing. First, provide attunement and openness to stay in the felt state while also permitting the child to move through by joining the child in how the body experiences and chooses to express this "pain." The felt "pain" location allows the child/client to identify where the experience occurs in the body. Invite them to outline/trace (in their mind or with their hand) around the described area. The movement invitation allows for the transformative experience of therapeutic integration.*

Vignette 2: The Turtle

> *"He doesn't want to talk or do anything. He seems anxious."*
> – Father of Justin, age 5

Five-year-old Justin was sitting in his hospital bed, holding his arms across his chest, his head down and a frown on his face. His parents communicated his lack of interest in playing or speaking to others.

I noticed his foot tapping in place. I began to tap my foot with his. "Let's start off like our feet," I told him, "And see if we can pretend to see where we would go." As we did this, we looked as if we were walking together in place. We agreed to take a journey with our bodies, and he expressed a desire to pretend to go "to the water." In response, we increased our movements and started to imitate swimming, moving our legs, arms, and heads like we were in the water.

Justin then stopped and pretended to be floating. He stated, "I am a turtle." As we moved like turtles, I noted to him that he had a protective shell and could peek out his head and explore when he wanted, on his own time. He then led me around the room, peeking out, looking at the various medical instruments and areas in the space. We took turns leading and following as we moved through the room. We moved slowly at first, eventually making the choice to increase our speed and more playfully become acquainted with the room.

What was so inspiring about this session was how, with the support to move, Justin came up with the idea of being a turtle, expressing the type of movement that enabled him to feel safe and comfortable and to get used to his environment. The use of movement permitted him to gain control over his body and advocate for his own timing and exploration of his surroundings. He transformed his anxiety-inducing state into a feeling of ease.

Vignette 2 Intervention: The Turtle

Activity Prompt: Use the following questions to explore with the child during your direct sessions: What animal would you like to be when you enter a new *environment*? How does that animal move through *the room (space)*? How are you similar or different from this animal? What does it *feel* like to move like this animal (i.e., help them to describe the felt sense)?

Provider Note: *The word space indicates the area around the child/individual, including the felt space within the body, between parts of the body, and outside the body between the child's body in relation to the environment, objects, and you, the provider. The space can be occupied by the child by moving directly from one point to another or around to occupy the entire kinesthetic area. You can describe the space as the environment the child is experiencing in his/her/their life: school, home, community, or even their own body. Pay attention to your observation of how the child's choices relate to their own state or psychological needs. Be sure to provide time to return to their original form – i.e., shaking off the movement experience, breathing, or tapping the body to reset. Remember that the word "feeling" indicates more than just emotional states (happy/sad, etc.) but rather the felt sense of the experience (i.e., difficulties, ease, discomforts, familiarities, or disconnects) as well as texture, temperature, and sensation.*

Vignette 3: Surviving the Volcano

"I am so uncomfortable when I have to wait! I feel bored. I hate it. There is nothing to do and no one understands."

– Jon, age 6

Jon's parents were concerned about his frustration and the "big feelings" that he displayed when he had to wait, didn't have a friend over, or a direct plan. His parents would solve his dilemmas immediately and give in to his requests, feeling their own annoyance over his perseverative words and so-called aggressive tone and behaviors. Each time they attempted to keep the peace, this unfortunately did not provide Jon with an opportunity to recognize his choices and increase his tolerance of frustration.

In our sessions, I supported Jon to sit in this discomfort and realize that his feelings were "his choice." Jon was given a metaphoric flashlight to see how his body held his discomfort: he noticed his furrowed brow, stomping feet, and quickened voice. At any moment he could decide how to use his time, manage his frustration, and change his posture or movements to ultimately engage with others. This took the shape of us going on our first journey using our imaginations. I asked Jon where he would like to go.

He decided to take us to the top of a volcano. He described it as hot, dangerous, and very uncomfortable for our bodies, tightening his muscles and squeezing into small areas around the imaginary volcano. We peeked into the volcano and moved quickly around it; he even attempted to touch it. Then we got stuck and were trapped without many options; he stood frozen in space with his hands held above his head, as if being restrained. I supported Jon's ability to problem-solve by amplifying his state of tension, mirroring for him the extreme place he had chosen to explore. Then, Jon said, "Let's put on volcano protective gear," using his imagination to create an adaptive alternative to being stuck. He was then able to end the movement journey by lowering his arms and firmly pressing his hands together. He brought contact to each part of his body as we patted out any remaining tension, and he then stood with a tall, confident stance.

Following our session, we explored how Jon was able to problem-solve and stay engaged even during his discomfort. He then expressed to me and his parents that he'd had the control and choice to solve his problem, also claiming to know how to get out of the toughest spots of an "actual volcano."

For the first time, Jon was able to stay in a nonpreferred state and feel his emotions, allowing him to figure out his solution. His parents felt relieved and understood that he was ready to tackle his challenges. They could join him and play along too.

Vignette 3 Intervention: **Surviving the Volcano**

Activity Prompt: Explore the following questions within your direct sessions with the child: What non-preferred feeling or difficult feeling have you had this week? Could you stay in it? Thinking back, now choose an image or a movement to express this feeling. How does the problem look now to you? Has it changed or is it different from your original feeling/experience? Can you share how long your feelings lasted?

Provider Note: You may verbally discuss the reflective questions in an observer role. The questions are intended to support the child/client to practice movement observation and embodied reflection throughout their daily interactions and to process states within the therapeutic environment. Encourage the child/client to move their body while reflecting on the events/feelings. Movement can look as simple as postural shifts, facial affect, or gross motor movements. Measuring the length (using a clock or counting) of emotion can support the individual to recognize that the feelings are transient and ever evolving versus being a definitive state or label. For example, a child may look at a jar of water and glitter. The feeling passes as the glitter floats from the top of a jar to the bottom.

Vignette 4: Riding the Bumps

> *"I always battle for control in my family. My six-year-old and I just argue all the time."*
>
> – Mother of Carla, age 6

Carla, a "willful" child, could independently dress herself, organize her colors, shapes, and even read. She was an amazing leader and helper to her friends, but at home with her mother, she had difficulty showing her strengths without a battle.

During one session, Carla and her mother shared with me a time when they were in the car and the road was very bumpy. Carla yelled at her mother that she was "too hot and it was too bumpy." As to be expected, Carla's mom felt overwhelmed by her daughter's discomfort. She wasn't intentionally making the car hot or the ride bumpy, but she was being yelled at for it.

I explored with Carla and her mother how to use a movement-based intervention. Given the awareness that Carla's response wasn't to be taken personally, her mother was encouraged to join Carla's movement, not her discomfort. Together we practiced by pretending we were in the car and explored how to rock more with the bumps. We even felt the wind blowing through the pretend windows to cool us down.

When Carla yelled, "Mom, it's too bumpy," her mother responded, "I agree. It's bumpy! Watch me bounce." Carla laughed, and together they rode the bumps until they figured out how to take control of the uncomfortable situation and find relief. This intervention helped to establish that each had different feelings, neither one of them had caused the problem (the heat, the bumps), and they could instead share the emotional load by being together and moving to a resolution with shared control.

Vignette 4 Intervention: Riding the Bumps

Activity Prompt: Explore the following concepts during your direct child sessions, asking the child to identify the following themes: Think about a time you got yelled at for something you could not control. Write three ways to work through this challenge (how could you ride the bumps, climb the hill, eat what was on your plate). Move your body with the (provider/parent) simultaneously to conquer and role-play the scenarios.

Provider Note: *In this exploration, you will find ways to join a child's challenged experience by sharing their load in a safe and contained environment. Support the child by physically joining them in their exploration. Try moving with the same qualities (time, weight, space), dimensional planes, and the use of your senses. Encourage your client to find resolutions through words and more so by reenacting the various outcomes together through movement. Here you may emphasize weight (especially) force (as in lifting up with full weight to feel competent) and ease (lightly lifting the fork to your mouth to eat the food), acknowledging the connection between efforts and how to resolve a life challenge. Model timing (speeding up/slowing down) and use the room's entire space to explore these conflicts. The goal is not to create a product but rather to create a sense of joining the child and engaging in the process, supporting the child to have choices and experience being part of a team.*

Vignette 5: Recognizing the Subtitles

"I want a pool, a larger room, and a castle LEGO set."

– Cody, age 8

Cody's parents communicated that their son was aware of recent devastation and homes lost to fires near them in California, but he was still focused on what he didn't have. His parents were worried that he had his priorities mixed up.

Cody entered our session appearing eager (large, dilated pupils, quickened voice, and fidgety hands) to discuss what gifts he wanted for the holidays. He shared that his parents seemed annoyed by his incessant needs and dialogue pertaining to his "wants," but he was confused about why. The more upset his parents got, the more insistent he was to seek out a reward.

To Cody, asking for holiday gifts was both very important and scary. His eyes widened as he acknowledged how some kids/people didn't have toys and their other belongings anymore. For Cody, having a wish list was important, especially because he knew his belongings could be destroyed, disappear, and life could change. This was the first news of hardship in Cody's immediate world. Physically, he showed his fear and discomfort via nonverbal communication, while his words sounded like selfish requests, though they meant so much more.

This therapeutic session provided a place to explore Cody's fears and support his parents in looking past their son's words to focus on his emotional requests. This practice hones in on what I call the "subtitles" of the child's narrative. Like this example, the content is expressed as if in a different language, but underneath the words are the subtitles that translate to Cody's parents how he is feeling and why he is communicating such needs (i.e. "Will I have what makes me happy? Will I be happy? Will everything be the same as I have been told and experienced so far? Am I safe?").

I worked collaboratively with Cody's parents to recognize and better understand how their child's pleading could indicate a need for safety and security. Additionally, Cody and his parents took turns with movement to explore patterns that felt familiar (holding hands, walking, hugging, standing, etc.) and patterns that could change (jumping, twisting, falling, leaning, etc.). By playing out the various patterns of movement, they further embodied the experiences of both insecurity and security. In the end, they joined hands and sat close to one another in an affectionate, secure bond (hugging firmly). Cody recognized that he was fortunate to be safe in his home, with his family, and that his concerns were understood.

Vignette 5 Intervention: **Recognizing the Subtitles**

Activity Prompt: Ask the child during your session to explore the following experiences and questions: Write your verbal responses to parents, situations/tasks, or even teachers (this statement is typically your adverse reaction, i.e., "No, stop, I won't"). Then write the subtitles: What is the feeling you are conveying (underlying the phrase you are saying)? It is fine to have your provider/or parent write for you if needed. For instance, when I say "no" to my parents when we are leaving for dinner reservations, I actually mean to say, "Give me a minute I am just finishing talking with my friend on the phone."

Provider Note: *The focus here is on the underlying emotional theme the child is presenting. Emotions are displayed by the body and through movement. Observe facial expressions, timing, posture, and movement profile. Notice the movement patterns revealed each week in the child's body and through their movements. The child will present similar body postures and movements based on his/her/their emotional state. Observing these patterns gives you insight before any spoken words or discussion from the child and their family. The parent or provider can also work on this activity without a child present – to further notice meaningful connections underlying the verbal statements heard at home.*

Vignette 6: Is Halloween Scary or Sweet?

> *"I want to be a superhero, I want to be a superhero. . . . I want to be a puppy dog!"*
>
> – Thomas, age 7

During the Halloween season in the United States, families choose costumes, purchase and hand out candy, and often join in parades, among other traditions. Time and money are spent to create each costume and determine how best to wear it for trick or treating. In therapy sessions, parents of children who have an overwhelming response to this holiday seek support on how to handle the feelings of their children. For example, why do children ruminate over a costume and then change their mind at the last minute? Why are there so many "big feelings" between parents and children during this time?

I started working with Thomas in October. His parents told me that he was very enthusiastic about the upcoming Halloween. Each year, he loved making choices about his costume, presents, and candy, etc. But then, they explained, as soon as they got excited with him and it got close to the actual holiday, he would change his mind and get upset. It seemed like the celebration of Halloween would be ruined.

With therapeutic support, we collaborated to understand how stress is experienced in the brain and how disruptive-movement patterns, such as increased speed when excited, rushing around when overwhelmed, hiding when scared, or even our physical response to the changes of a few late nights and increased sugar, can be challenging for any child and parent to normalize.

Thomas's parents were relieved to learn that their son's feelings were valid due to the increased changes he experienced during the Halloween season. In choosing a costume he was trying to gain control, yet he was also overwhelmed. With therapeutic support, he communicated what he was feeling; he noted that the weather had changed and gotten colder; his school schedule had become less structured with more assemblies, decorations, and lots of noise; even his own home and neighborhood looked different. He pointed out that on Halloween, he also faced large crowds at school (with parents taking photos), and strangers arrived at the door of his home. To him this was very unusual and caused discomfort.

Thomas found relief as he explored with his parents how to anticipate and gain more control during the Halloween season. They created a visual calendar to count down the days, they communicated with his teacher about options for participation, and they even mapped out the route for trick or treating.

I worked with Thomas and his parents to practice Halloween-related movement and role playing. He would pretend to be wearing the costume he had chosen, ultimately deciding what felt best in his body (standing tall like a superhero, flying, and saving the day or crawling, barking, and moving like a dog). By embodying these choices Thomas was able to stick with a decision. The family also practiced making noises, surprising one another (moving fast/slow), and problem-solving for any unexpected moments. Thomas's parents realized that it was much easier to set him up for success by playing out scenarios, moving through them, and planning with him.

Vignette 6 Intervention: **Is Halloween Scary or Sweet?**

Activity Prompt: Use the following prompt to support the child during the one-to-one sessions or group sessions: Practice acting out an experience that may be challenging. Explore with movement the anticipated worries.

Provider Note: *Help the child identify the "what if's" and "oh no's," within their thinking and decision-making. First, explore the psychoeducation question, "What does the brain look like during stress, and how does it work?" Then, ask, "How do we recognize what a child needs by looking at the body?" and "How can we move and embody this experience so that a new pattern emerges?" You can explore these experiences with the whole family, individual clients, or within your progress notes.*

Vignette 7: Are You Full of Thanks?

"It's hard to be thankful. I don't understand what's happening."
— Carlton, age 6

Because of his parents' separation, Carlton would now be spending Thanksgiving in two different homes. He was doing well in school but made little to no eye contact when someone talked to him, appeared lethargic and withdrawn, and had difficulty talking about his feelings. Carlton was confused about the changes in his family life and had a limited sense of self-compassion; he didn't feel good about himself. Therapy helped clarify the changes he was experiencing and provided an environment for building a sense of his own strengths. By acknowledging his own worth and capabilities, Carlton found ways to cope and assert himself to get his needs met with his family.

We worked together to explore his "truths," such as what did he notice about his body, his senses, his movements? In the therapeutic session, Carlton explored how his feet could hold his body, how he could control his speed, and the many ways his body could move (jumping, turning, pushing, pulling). He realized that he had control over his actions and thoughts. He communicated thankfulness for his ability to move and express his feelings using his entire body. He developed an awareness of his senses, listened longer, watched his surroundings, and explored those abilities.

Carlton has since taken his new awareness into his two homes and shared his personal thanks. This year on Thanksgiving, Carlton said, he plans to share with his family who he is and what he can do.

Vignette 7 Intervention: Are You Full of Thanks?

Activity Prompt: Share the following prompt within your therapeutic sessions: A helpful practice is showing gratitude and thankfulness for what you have and who you are. One way to know if you are full of thanks is by exploring what is absolutely true. Think, discuss, and write about what you know your body can do. For instance, what do your feet do, what do your hands hold? What do you hear, see, and feel? Etc.

Provider Note: *This is a sensory mindfulness exercise to be used within the child's one-on-one or family session. Helping the child reflect on what is true for them can ease anxiety. Truths can be the senses you can see, feel, hear, touch, taste, and physically move. For instance, the child knows he can hear the sound of a bird or the feeling of his soft blanket. A child can know she is moving her arm or tasting a sweet apple. Try to explore by slowing down, naming each sense, and using the body to take in the information thoroughly.*

Vignette 8: Reduce Stress

> *"What if I don't get better? What if I have to have more procedures, tests, and checkups? What if I miss more classes and more time with friends?"*
>
> – Sarah, age 10

When I met Sarah, she immediately started talking about her worries. She anticipated all the worst scenarios and outcomes. Right away I noticed a disconnect between what she said and what her posture revealed. While her words were filled with anxiety, her facial affect was flat, her breathing was steady, and her body was seated upward in her chair. She appeared detached from her statements, as if she was reciting a script she had said over and over to anyone who confronted her.

We took this opportunity to gain more knowledge about her physicality. How did these anticipatory thoughts feel in her body? Where did she hold these feelings? Instantly, she slouched over, seeming to be weighted down. We decided to explore various postures that felt heavy, as if we were being pressed downward. As we practiced pushing, we talked about the pressures of having an illness, various negative experiences, and the unknown. We also realized that the tension in our postures felt quite strong and powerful.

Sarah took a step forward and pushed up toward the sky with her hands. She pressed down on the heels of her feet and stood tall. She recognized that her worries also presented opportunities to be brave that could lead to positive outcomes. Her vulnerability could lead to strength and growth.

We then took on new powerful poses and movements, adding breathing exercises and even smiles. Sarah was able to transform her discomfort (those pressures) and repetitive thoughts into adaptive experiences from which she could learn.

Her tight composure inhibited her ability to connect with others and navigate new experiences. The experience of more freedom in her body through movement allowed Sarah to be vulnerable and be met with a mirroring of strength and ease. Additionally, the space for therapeutic movement allowed for a stronger relational bond with the therapist and helped her move toward connection to her emotional past and ultimately recovery.

Vignette 8 Intervention: **Reduce Stress**

Activity Prompt: Use the following prompt to explore movement within your clinical sessions: Start by writing down moments/experiences where you had to move with different qualities of weight (heaviness – lifting a heavy brick or feeling pressure from too much/lightness – lifting a simple feather or celebrating the end of the school day). Can you make that posture? Do you feel the strength in your body? Explore shifting the direction of the pose. What do you recognize or feel now?

Provider Note: *Notice your weightedness while observing and mirroring the child's posture/movements. Remember, there are no mistakes. Model movement postures that support increased use of weight. Asking questions, noticing facial expressions, the length of time the child can hold the pose, and the ease/discomfort of shifting that posture in the session. You can support the child by writing for them or asking the questions and giving examples to support their dialogue.*

Vignette 9: Goodbye Anxiety

"I don't like meeting new friends or entering new places."

– Willa, age 15

Willa's anxiety caused her to avoid new environments and develop compulsive habits that led her to pull out her hair (clinically known as trichotillomania). In her treatment facility, she avoided talking and engaging with others, yet she was interested in movement. "When I move, I feel like I have control; my mind is clear. I feel so comfortable," she said.

I asked her to use movement to define and think about her anxiety. How did it look? How did it move? In our initial session, Willa leaned steadily and rocked from side to side. However, every time she attempted to shift her focus toward the ceiling, extend her reach upward, or rise to a standing position, she promptly halted herself and resumed her preferred side-to-side movements. It seemed as though there was a pressure constraining her. She persistently attempted this vertical motion (aiming to ascend or reach up) on multiple occasions during the session but never surpassed the height of her shoulders. She looked like a little child reaching up but not high enough to get the cookies off a shelf.

Willa shared memories of not being allowed to perform a task in her home such as getting her own food. Within the therapy sessions, she was now able to assert herself. She reached her arms up above her head and lengthened them toward the sky to demonstrate her feelings. She ended the session by drawing a picture of herself entering a new environment. She expressed her awareness of her potential and claimed to feel safe and secure in her body and abilities.

Willa's treatment center felt the need to enlist my services with the hopes of advancing her progress. She had shared an interest in body-centered work versus solely talk therapy. She trusted in the center's recommendation, which laid the foundation for our therapeutic relationship. What had taken the center months to unravel (stopping her destructive behaviors and avoidant/withdrawing communication) took moments within Willa's first fifty-minute therapeutic dance/movement therapy session. Her body had been holding and demonstrating her "tearing out" feeling, manifested in her destructive behaviors, but she now permitted herself to release this tension and reclaim her independence.

Vignette 9 Intervention: **Goodbye Anxiety?**

Activity Prompt: Continue to use the following prompt to explore movement within your clinical sessions: Let's explore the movement planes in order to rid yourself of that anxious feeling. Start by moving side to side in the horizontal plane for soothing and ease. Now shift and move vertically with a sense of ego and confidence. Now move sagittally to connect with someone in the room or the environment. Did you have a preferred plane of movement? Write down what you notice.

Provider Note: *Emulate the child's experience of moving through the planes: soothing horizontal, standing securely in the world for the first time, or moving with one another for connection. Moving in the dimensional planes can be done with the entire body or just one body part (arms, head, legs, finger). Notice, discuss, and document the preferences as an assessment tool to reveal psychological patterns and understand how the child moves in the given situation or where to provide interventions.*

Vignette 10: Is My Child Acting With Aggression?

> *"Be careful. She hits and breaks things. She is very aggressive."*
> – Caregiver of Audrey, age 9

When I walked into the room, nine-year-old Audrey lunged toward me with her arms outstretched and her fist moving directly at my shoulder to make contact. It appeared to her family that she was trying to punch me;

they gasped and told me, "Look out!" But I acknowledged and observed in Audrey's action the quality of sustained lightness in her movement from her elbow down to her fist. While she had limited words and presented with neurodivergence, I knew it was important to understand what her body communicated.

For me, the qualities of Audrey's movement were not meant to be hurtful; rather, she had just been saying hello. She was making contact and ensuring that she would touch me before I could have an opportunity to reach or move her. I had no intention of doing that, but that had been her experience with most other adults.

When I didn't shudder, frown, yell, or pull away, Audrey smiled. She put her arm down and stood looking at me. She began to sway. She moved side to side in a soothing, rocking rhythm. I responded verbally and followed with my own body in a rhythm much like a heartbeat. I acknowledged to Audrey that I admired her way of soothing and caring for herself. She moved toward a stuffed animal, picked it up, and began to rock the toy in place.

Several times in my exchanges with Audrey, she would move toward someone or something with what was perceived as pressure or aggression. Every time, I empowered the adults to see her need to feel her own body, to find security, and to connect. When we initiated movement with input such as joint compression, rhythmic motion, or collaborative movement, she would comply, soften, and appear to engage appropriately.

The perceived threats of Audrey's direct, quick movements had limited her relationships and kept others far away, fearful. She now had new ways to be understood. She could move and find support without needing to lunge at others in an attempt to protect herself. Adults started speaking to her *before* making contact and modeling other options for her to connect.

Vignette 10 Intervention: Is My Child Acting With Aggression?

Activity Prompt: Model for the child's parents and practice the following movement-based exercise. Use the following prompt for the child to explore this activity: Have the provider or parent take each of your fingers and press (safely/firmly) into the joints where your fingers connect. Imagine giving the joints a hug or a squeeze. Repeat this on each finger. Have the provider/parent move to the wrist, arm, and shoulder. Continue doing this to feet, ankle bone, and knee. Explore the type of pressure that feels grounding and safe.

Provider Note: *This is similar to joint compression/tactile input to support regulation and increased attentional focus. Incorporate the breath between and during physical input to allow for co-regulation and activation of the parasympathetic nervous system. Remember that identifying input preferences allows for appropriate relational touch, helping the child feel a safe connection, and introduces self-regulation tools for the child. As you explore this activity do you notice increased attention or mood stability in the child?*

Vignette 11: Can You Hear the Body?

"I have constant pain. I am especially uncomfortable when I am surrounded by doctors asking me questions, and the unknown prognosis of my illness."

– Kata, age 14

When I met Kata, she identified pain in her head and stomach. Curious, I engaged her in dialogue to learn about her preferred activities. I sat at eye level with her while she initiated talking about her favorite television shows. I wanted to create a safe space for her to feel she could be in control and choose what to speak about. She said of her favorite TV show, "I love knowing the characters in a show and feeling connected." Based on this, I knew that bonding with her would significantly support her ease during her hospitalization.

Then Kata immediately showed tension in her body when her medical team walked in the room and began to discuss her pain. The more people surrounded her, the more her body tensed up. Her voice grew quiet, and she picked at her bracelet as if to dig her way out of the situation. Her pain, from my perspective, shifted from physical to psychological. She was scared and vulnerable.

After Kata's team had departed, I narrated my observation of her body language and movements. She looked at me with tear-filled eyes and stated, "I have to protect myself." We explored whether she felt there was a purpose to her pain (did it serve any benefit to her?).

I provided a therapeutic "container" for Kata to safely consider her discomfort by joining me in a movement exploration. I had her identify what her pain felt like, looked like, and, most importantly, how it moved. She described her pain as "slime," a toy popular with teens. This slime was "yucky" and filled her head. She described it further and moved her body as if she were overpowered by this "gooey substance," rocking side to side as if pouring the slime upside down. I had her trace the line of her pain (where the feeling started and stopped): The pain poured from her head down her shoulders to her stomach.

As Kata became aware of the somatization of this pain, she was able to rephrase her description of pain from messy to a protective coating, the gooey sense of having an extra layer of skin to shield her. As soon as she embodied this insight and physical change, she released her posture, regulated her breathing, and appeared at ease.

Afterward Kata looked at me and asked, "How do I do this alone?" She wanted to know what to do after the session when I, the therapist, would not be with her. We reviewed the steps using the acronym, DANCE.

- Differentiating her movements and feelings
- Attaching them together with a theme
- Narrating her experience
- Consciously connecting to one another by moving
- Engaging her choice to find ease (empathically)

Kata saw how her body had the wisdom to shield her when needed. Rather than become detached and upset, she now had access to leaning in and feeling safe. She was enthusiastic about having new options to support her anxiety and pain and appreciated me for recognizing and "hearing her body."

Vignette 11 Intervention: Can You Hear the Body?

Activity Prompt: Use the following prompt within the clinical session. Invite the child to try the following activity: Try to DANCE with your family/or the provider. D: Identify a precise movement. A: Keep moving to expand from one part of the body to the whole body (i.e., a phrase of movement/routine, multiple movements). Explore the movement theme. What is the feeling? N: Verbally state and communicate more about the situation or feeling. C: Join with your family to try each other's movement phrases, bringing to consciousness. E: empathically engage the many options to stay in or shift out of the state nonverbally and verbally.

> **Provider Note:** *D: Differentiate; A: Attach; N: Narrate; C: Consciousness; E: Empathic engagement. This exploration can be done by the child or with the child in which you, the provider, communicate verbally the DANCE that is being expressed in each step of the interaction. This movement exploration starts from single movements of one part of the body and expands to the child using the entire body. You, the provider, bring words to what you are witnessing and awareness to help the child connect the whole experience. You are supporting the experience of being seen and supporting through movement with therapeutic attunement. The narration of the child's movements will accurately depict what is happening versus a labeled judgement or inaccurate emotional label. Use words based on the actual movements you see, (i.e., your hand is moving forward instead of you are rushing; your mouth is frowning instead of you are sad). Children can feel a vast range of emotions at the same time, feeling confused, hungry, curious, comfortable, silly, and even annoyed. Labeling the movement creates more accuracy for awareness, resilience, and connection.*

Vignette 12: Careless or Carefree?

> *"What are we doing? What are we doing . . . today? Where are we going?"*
> — Peter, age 5

Summer brings with it extra time and opportunities to explore during long, carefree days and to connect with friends. But what if, during this time, your child seems to have more meltdowns and appears more disorganized and needy?

Peter communicated his excitement for summer. He smiled and jumped up and down when he talked about swimming at the pool. Naturally, his parents assumed this meant he loved swimming and that they didn't have to think much more about plans for summer because long days at the pool would do the trick.

While children can show enjoyment by smiling and jumping, other movements may depict tension, anxiety, and dysregulation. Peter's perseverative behaviors, including incessant questions and an urgency to move from one task to the next, indicated his lack of ease. He appeared never to be satiated. His eyes darted back and forth, his hands flapped, and he paced about the room. With further observation, even his facial expression appeared strained versus happy and excited.

We worked collaboratively to create a visual summer schedule that supported balanced summer days and offered activities both energetic and relaxing. This schedule was different from his secure routine during the school year, so Peter needed support to understand the many transitions he would experience in the coming days.

We played with movement experiences to practice slowing down and explored reading each other's nonverbal cues, facial expressions, and gestures. Peter's parents identified the frequency (how often he stated a new request versus his ability to sustain attention on a given task) and duration (how long he could appear fulfilled in an interaction) of his excitement and learned strategies to support regulation across environments: for instance, how to anticipate when a game of tag is over and it's time to transition into the classroom or how to know when a peer is done with a toy or needs more space. We also determined how to accept feelings that may arise when plans change or when he needs extra space (independence from others, larger environments rather than intimate playrooms).

Vignette 12 Intervention: Careless or Carefree?

Activity Prompt: To switch the focus from "careless" (a lack of organization or ease) to a carefree state (sequences and ease), invite the child or family to explore the following tasks: To create a sensory schedule, think about the five senses. List five tasks or activities you will do throughout your day. For instance, for the sense of hearing (sounds): I will listen to an audiobook or nature sounds. For the sense of sight: go on a nature hunt. Next, for the sense of taste: Enjoy a meal with your family. And for the sense of touch: Explore textures of clothes and stuffed animals. Identify the order in which these sensory tasks would provide for a feeling of ease and help to organize the day for the child and/or the family. Invite the child/parent to try the order during the upcoming days/week and report back at the following session.

Provider Note: *The sensory schedule allows for an easy flow during morning, day, and night transitions and builds the child's awareness about whether they approach the specific task/activity with a careless or carefree nature. You can change the order if the child presents with increased resistance or if the family requests a change. Increase the range of ideas to promote expanded coping skills and a "larger tool kit" of integrative skills for the child. Take note that the sensory diet can support organization and overall emotional regulation. You are encouraged to keep trying options of sensory activities and different orders of the activities with the family until they report more of a flow during their days.*

Vignette 13: Shedding Light on Comfort

"She is really anxious around people."

– Mother of Lucy, age 4

Every time Lucy had a medical procedure, a visitor, or a change in her hospital environment, she became upset, withdrawing herself from the people around her. During one encounter, she sat alone in her room under blankets, her arms crossed and only her eyes directed at me. I decided to use our sensory system to create an experience that would improve her comfort level and provide her with a sense of control – to transform her enlarged view of the unknown, an environment out of her control, into a subtler, softer space within her "reachability" (an activity that would involve only the use of her eyes). I took the flashlight next to her bed (typically used by the doctors) and started to explore the surroundings. I created a pattern in which I moved the light slowly to a spot, stopped, and then moved it away. Lucy smiled, following the light with her eyes as the pattern continued; she was anticipating the light's next movement.

I shifted the light to our bodies, where I shined it directly on Lucy's arms and feet and then on mine. Next, I put the light down, and we continued to generate ideas and move together.

Vignette 13 Intervention: Shedding Light on Comfort

Activity Prompt: Use the following activity prompt in your therapeutic sessions or provide as an activity for the child to explore at home with family: Flashlight play – Take a flashlight to a safe space (a familiar environment like your bedroom, the therapy room, or a preferred room in your house where you feel you have the freedom to explore and where you are surrounded by objects and images you feel comfortable around) and explore materials, items, and your body in this space. Shine the light on different areas as you explore (for example: What do you see in the room? What do you notice you are wearing? What do you notice about different parts of your body, fingers, or toes?). Evoke movement with the light by changing the speed at which you discover new places or changing the timing of turning off and on the light. Notice the differences that emerge when the light is close or far away.

> **Provider Note:** *The light allows the visual system to zoom in and out and adjust to the various visuals in the room or on the child's body. The light can support comfort in minimizing distractions and increasing focus on one point at a time. Ensure your client anticipates what will happen next, take turns taking leadership of the light, support safety by identifying what is in the room first, and how to safely communicate if/when the lights in the room need to be turned back on or stay on. This activity can take a few moments or can be done throughout an entire session.*

By acknowledging Lucy's need for control, I gave her an awareness of her vision, which I called her "natural superpower." With this superpower, she could use her eyes to look around, explore, and anticipate who would be near her and what was happening. We continued to use this as a tool in other interactions. She became more comfortable with moments she could not control. She even initiated holding our flashlight and sharing with me and others all the things she could see.

Vignette 14: Regulation, Communication, Integration, Oh My!

> *"Mommy, where are you going? One more hug, one more kiss . . . What are you doing? How? When?"*
>
> – Patricia, age 6

Often parents wonder what is age appropriate. What is "normal" for a child? When Patricia came to my office, her parents expressed concerns about her lack of interest in playing with others and her increased tendency to pick her fingernails and hold her body in a strained position whenever they separated from her. They communicated her distress when she encountered a new environment or a change of plans.

Upon meeting Patricia, I immediately saw that she walked hesitantly, stiff behind her mother's legs, and then she sat with her legs in a "W" position (a common physical pattern observed in children with poor core stability, which impacts breathing, eye contact, and focus). Her hands twisted inward, and her fingers grasped nothing.

Interestingly, Patricia had already received ten months of verbal therapy focused on her anxious feelings, and she had learned words to describe emotions, such as "I feel scared." Yet her body did not present with ease and comfort (not in fluid motion, nor calm and alert), which left her with outstanding questions, insecurities, and challenges, both physically and socially.

When Patricia was given an opportunity to explore her sensory preferences and discover how to perceive and embody her environment through more adaptive integrated movement, a change occurred. The therapeutic sessions supported her in learning about her superpower: How she could use her sense of touch to feel connected and supported before entering a visually stimulating environment, thus providing input to her body through movement and physical contact with her parents before an event. I guided Patricia and her mom to stand in front of each other, then reach hand to hand, to identify self and other and to establish Patricia's understanding of her body boundaries.

Additionally, Patricia was encouraged to sit in a more grounded posture rather than the "W" position, by using the weight of her hands to display intentional control of her movements. She became increasingly more comfortable, sitting upright, making clearer eye contact, and communicating with more words. She was able to practice entering environments to prime herself for more to come.

Her parents learned about using "inclusion" words, such as "join" instead of "help." For instance, her mom joined her by playfully speaking and walking her into school versus helping her by carrying her into the classroom. Her parents anticipated her questions, spoke directly to her, and fostered her independence and self-compassion. For example, her parents got down at her eye level and said, "You are going into school, and you will see your teacher, now you can march or hop into the doorway. I admire your bright smile today!"

This embodied lens and action-based language, (e.g., how the child is moving), provided a more integrated path toward Patricia's autonomy.

Vignette 14 Intervention: Regulation, Communication, Integration, Oh, My!

Activity Prompt: Use the following prompt within your clinical session or to share as an activity for the child to do at home with family: Find your body boundaries by exploring where your body starts and physically stops. Trace with your finger around your body, either laying on the ground (switching hands to reach each part) or standing up and use a mirror or partner to help while tracing your body boundaries.

Provider Note: *Model and practice breathing together while tracing the child's body. Help the child notice where there is physical skin/bones/muscle space versus negative space (the area around the body not touching them). Support the child to slow down while tracing. You can physically indicate boundaries by having the child lie down on a large piece of paper using colored pencils to trace the child's body. You can also trace an imaginary line that is just felt and explored. Discuss what boundaries are essential to the child including what their emotional limits and physical limitations are. Use the wall, floor, and even your body to support the awareness of self versus others. For example, pressing on the wall versus reaching out in front towards the open space.*

Vignette 15: Are You a Super Flyer?

"Are we there yet?"

– Thomas, age 2

When Thomas was two years old, his parents decided to travel to the East Coast via airplane for their first trip across the country. They sought out my professional expertise for taking child development to new heights and parenting to the skies – from my book *Super Flyers: A Parent Guidebook for Airplane Travel with Children*. We discussed their plans to have the most success: Ease in packing, comfort in travel, and the knowledge required to get through it (Baudino, 2017). We discussed their biggest worries: What if he doesn't sit still on the plane? What if he makes a ton of noise? What if we forget things and we are stuck on the plane without what we need? One of the initial concepts I shared is my acronym, A.H.H., a thoughtful and embodied way to prepare for any transition, in this case, the airplane (Baudino, 2017, pp. 10–13).

We explored the "A.H.H." of preparing for the flight. Aim to get everything packed and ready twenty-four hours before the flight. That way, the day of travel is dedicated to playing, relaxing, and keeping up the normal routine. This allows parents to have successful transitions and to stay present with their children. Humor applies to softening expectations. Be flexible, stay positive, and make it fun. Thomas's parents discussed ways to share their roles and to be available during potential situations that could occur on the flight. Happiness was explored by giving Thomas opportunities to role-play how to act appropriately on the airplane. He practiced controlling his tone of voice, options for movement within the cabin, and finding areas to explore. He was able to look at pictures, ask questions, and work out his feelings about traveling with his parents. Thomas and his family learned the importance of being aware of their individual needs and emotions related to flying, which led to acceptance for the journey ahead.

Vignette 15 Intervention: Are You a Super Flyer?

Activity Prompt: Share this activity prompt with the child and family you are working with in the clinical session for their next travel experiences with their family: Practice the acronym A.H.H. with your parent or provider —**A**im to get everything packed before 24 hours of the flight; **H**umor: Be flexible, stay positive, and make it fun with your expectations; and **H**appiness: Role-play and act out scenarios to practice what it's like to be on a plane (tone of voice, how to move, and how to keep entertained).

Provider Note: *Explore the A.H.H. with the child and their family before traveling, including planes, road trips, trains, and more. Emphasize the importance of moving and role-playing in addition to talking.*

Vignette 16: The Importance of Being Aware

> *"She is so scared, uncomfortable, and overwhelmed she doesn't want to do anything. She hasn't even smiled."*
>
> – Father of Kaitlyn, age 8

Intense pain, discomfort, or stress is often very difficult to change. Some people recommend finding distractions, but in my therapeutic work, I believe in empowerment.

Kaitlyn was so overwhelmed by her physical and emotional experiences of having a medical illness and her new surroundings at the hospital. She wouldn't move, speak, or show interest in interacting with others. She appeared frightened by anyone who even came close to her. I observed her sitting in a curled-up position with her arms wrapped tightly around her knees. I felt a longing to support her in this state while creating the opportunity for her to experience the reality of the here and now and a chance for a playful and safe exchange with her father.

I told Kaitlyn about her super senses – her abilities to interact in her own time. She didn't have to interact with me yet; she only needed to use her own senses. In our therapeutic session, I prompted her to start by listening to three different sounds in the room. When she began to listen, I noticed her loosen her grip on her knees. Next, I invited her to look for two different shapes. I witnessed her eyes gaze upward and focus on the ceiling. Her posture shifted and her knees fell open into a relaxed, seated position. Lastly, I asked her to become aware of the sensations felt on or in her body, heat, cold air, soft cotton clothes, her skin, and her own hair. She looked me in the eye and communicated that her discomfort had ceased. Kaitlyn then allowed her father to wrap his arms around and rock her. They joined hands and started to play and move together; they heard more sounds, explored more sights, and expressed more joy.

Vignette 16 Intervention: The Importance of Being Aware

Activity Prompt: Explore the following concepts by asking the child to complete the following tasks: Tune into what you see, hear, and feel. Practice noticing your surroundings by using your senses. Count together how many sounds you hear, colors you see, and the textures/feelings experienced on the body (soft, cold, itchy). Explore your emotions and the themes you see/feel in the room (i.e., asking is there a serious tone or a silly tone in your interaction?).

Provider Note: *Support parents to practice tuning in with their child. Help the parent and child get a baseline of the environment and any noticed changes. Support using the senses and these awareness skills for everyday transitions and waiting moments. Provide opportunities for the child to become a detective (of their feelings and themes) and fully be present and aware. Utilizing the senses can help to understand and gain control of one's choices.*

Vignette 17: To Distinguish, Not Diagnose

"Oh, I guess I am okay."

– David, age 10

David had experienced physical and mental challenges throughout his life. Although he wasn't very talkative, he was observant of others and always wore a smile. His posture, however, was stiff, as if there was heaviness in his body. His father acted noticeably stressed and worried in front of David.

He wept when he spoke about his son's challenges, but smiled at his son and asked him to put on a brave face.

Like most parents, David's father had an easier time when observing his son having fun and laughing; however, this session enabled David to link his body actions to the vast range of his emotions and to allow him to share with his father his actual feelings whether challenging or positive. We started by moving and acknowledging David's posture, speed, and motion. David communicated that he felt sad. We expanded and linked his movements together. I encouraged him to accept his feelings, and he responded by moving vertically. His hands reached up, and he bobbed his head up and down. We talked about how it felt to be aware of his own choices through his actions. I invited him to move his body, shifting forward and back, as if we were playing catch, as he shared things that made him feel sad. He began to move more quickly, perhaps to push his sad feelings away. But finally, he softened and sat up, took a deep breath, and lowered his body into the chair. He stated he felt better. He had never been allowed to feel the full extent of his emotions. He communicated that it would feel bad to have others see him sad; he "wouldn't want to make someone feel worse." I observed that just by using his body to experience his feelings, he was able to make a shift on his own, for his own comfort and happiness.

The therapeutic support here fostered a better understanding and acceptance of David's daily challenges, feelings, and social relationships. Having a place to express and witness these feelings with his father created validation and a healthy connection.

Vignette 17 Intervention: To Distinguish, Not Diagnose

Activity Prompt: The following activity is provided to support attunement and emotional regulation. Invite the child to participate in the following tasks/requests: First, your parent or provider will match your eye level (so they are nonthreatening and connected to you), then instead of reacting to your emotion they will join you in the challenge of that emotion you are displaying. For instance, if you are frustrated, your parent or provider would explore making their movements like yours however amplifying the way they move. This could look like, for example, stomping your feet and your parent/provider stomping bigger to overemphasize the feeling you are exhibiting. Alternatively, your parent/provider could soften their stomp and make your emotional display seem smaller and less upsetting. You may also explore making your movement reactions bigger or smaller (amplify versus minimize). Notice how this sharing of the emotional load supports you to feel seen and supported.

Provider Note: *Remember to encourage and model empathy and curiosity. The interaction does not look like mockery or mimicking. The emphasis on the body allows the child to reflect and share their emotional load. Have the child explore both positive and negative feelings. Use one part of the body or the entire body (i.e., the child stomps his feet, and the adult throws down her fist; the child lays on the floor, and the provider sits on the chair).*

Reference

Baudino, L. (2017). *Super Flyers: A parent guidebook for airplane travel with children.* CreateSpace Independent Publishing Platform.

Chapter 2

The Therapeutic Lens Explored

Critical Areas in Children – Anxiety and Pain

Whether the moving moment vignette conveyed the story of a child presenting with anxiety, chronic pain disorders, emotional dysregulation, or neurodivergence, the treatment was individualized, with clear and consistent principles identified through the lens of dance/movement therapy. The sessions provided therapeutic support by bringing awareness to body movements, sensations, and intentions while using play, connection, and embodied attunement between the child, therapist, and family members.

Anxiety

Anxiety is one of the most prevalent diagnoses given to patients (Lebrun-Harris, Ghandour, Kogan, & Warren, 2022). In various disorders, anxiety symptoms may exist due to medical, environmental, relational, and situational contexts. The child with anxiety responds to perceived or actual fear and the anticipation of future threats. As a result, the presentation of the reaction indicates a functional disturbance or may hinder or otherwise impact daily interactions, experiences, and relationships. Illness and disorder are identified by criteria/symptoms and based on frequency, duration, and situational context; however, anxiety states may also be adaptive and part of normal functioning.

I have observed firsthand that many children with displayed anxiety also experience sensory integration challenges and differences throughout their development. A primary focus of my work, and this book, is to discuss this link between the predisposition to anxiety, the body, and the sensory system. Similarly, research on the sensory system, dating back to the 1970s with Jean Ayres's work, points to the compounding factors of environment and nervous system responses to a child's relationships in the world (Ayres & Robbins, 2005). When the body feels organized and supported, a child reveals a sense of calm and an alert state. The child's body no longer presents a defensive or reactive response of fear or anxiety. The moving moment vignettes show that dance/movement therapy allows the body to receive input safely and further regulates the system with connection and communication.

DOI: 10.4324/9781003363491-3

Interestingly, in many of the therapeutic interactions provided in Chapter 1, the children had a parallel process not only to movement and their emotional regulation, but a deeper patterning that was shared with me in the parent intake regarding the child's birth story and early developmental interactions/relationships. During the intake process, parents and I find fascination in the similarities and nature of their child's birth story to their developmental character, challenges, and strengths. For example, the narratives of the baby's born by "flying" out of the birth canal, via C-section, or born two-weeks late, correspond with impatience or a ravenous thirst for learning, developmental delays or difficulty transitioning, respectively. These instances are not intended to assign blame or formulate assumptions but to bring awareness of the connection from birth through early development – the, I like to say, "consistently inconsistent" patterns. Furthermore, the holding of these patterns to be significant and meaningful allows the parent and provider insight into the signs and actions the child displays. This predictability in experience and action allows for an ease and containment of the relational triggers/responses. The parents' reflections and associations of their child's complete story (both consciously and unconsciously) serve as an unveiling in how the parents see and respond to their children. Hence, promoting a more thorough exploration of background and developmental history of the child contributes to further comprehension of the patterns of movement, disposition, and regulation, which can subsequently be acknowledged, correlated, and evolved.

To explain further, when an adult experiences the unpredictability of a child who is overwhelmed, this is typically due to the unknown feeling state, the randomness of the child's actions, and the adult's lack of insight. When children enter new growth stages, such as starting kindergarten or transitioning into third grade, it is important to return to their patterns from birth and early development for insight into their communication and behaviors. This can help us understand how they are adapting to their new environment and what they may need from us. The historical review of the child brings predictability to the interactions and clearer insight toward their body-based response to the sensory world around them.

Sensory Impact

I postulate that many children who exhibit anxiety may have an underlying sensory, body-based discrepancy, a neuroceptive gauge of stress that has impacted their sense of security, potentially from their very beginning. A threatened body presents as an anxious child. For instance, a child who shows early signs of stress at birth and throughout the early developmental ages, what doctors call "fussy, colic, withdrawn, or difficult," or has adverse responses to sounds, sights, and touch, is a child set with a highly dialed-up stress response.

Throughout a child's development, notice whether he/she/they has difficulty with changes in daily routines or completing simple tasks, such as changing clothes. Does the child have aversions or marked reactions to sounds (covering the ears), increasing noise, or pickiness in eating, sleeping, or toileting? These responses are adaptive choices the child has established as protection from the ongoing and constant threat experienced in their body. When the child's body undergoes a physiological danger, the body experiences opposition to the world, others, or the self. The child may then present with perseverative speaking by attempting to negotiate out of situations, repeating questions, delaying responses to expectations, presenting with ritualistic behaviors, and using unclear communication.

The anxious child needs a grounded, integrated container to support learning and development. The child's embodied anxiety will then be expressed verbally and with awareness of body states and needs. Simultaneously, the child may access the ability to think outside the box (an executive-functioning skill) and expand the creative mind to consider options versus omissions or avoidance tactics. As the threats diminish, the child becomes capable. This premise supports treating and understanding anxiety in children.

Therapeutic Lens

As I tell my clients, I rely on a top-down and bottom-up view of therapeutic support. Historically, medical, and psychological practices have focused on how the brain impacts an individual's social, emotional, and physical behaviors (Taylor, Goehler, Galper, et al., 2010). Treatment that identifies methods that foster talking, thinking, and problem-solving, to name a few, is considered a top-down approach. I look at how the brain (top-down) responds to stress and how the body (bottom-up) responds, holds, and expresses anxiety (Van Der Kolk, 2014). The brain and body react to anticipatory worries, identified as "what if" statements that contribute to the anxious state of mind and the body's presentation of movements and sensations in a reactive or threatened state (Homann, 2010).

When we look at how the brain responds to stress, research supports strategies that integrate connection between the primitive reptilian, lower-brain areas and the executive functioning, higher-brain, prefrontal cortex (Diamond, 2016). Regulation is created by breathing and moving within the body. The amygdala, the brain's emotion center, has close communication with the areas responsible for memory, attention, planning, and behavioral control (Farran, Miller, Kaufman, & Davis, 1997; Rolls, 1992; Schulkin, McEwen, & Gold, 1994; Cisler, 2017; Park, Leonard, Saxler, et al., 2018). Emotions are activated in the brain and the neuronal connections located in the "gut brain," which are then expressed through the body in search of well-being (Porges, 2022; Kolacz, Kovacic, & Porges, 2019). The gut brain is identified as the two-way communication between the nervous system, which allows for a pathway between the emotional and cognitive centers of the brain and throughout the body (Carabotti, Scirocco, Maselli, & Severi, 2015). This is exciting, as we physically feel emotions in our body and can recognize the body's communication flow upward to our thinking brain for building understanding, repair, and connection.

Dr. Stephen Porges's polyvagal theory identifies how our nervous system helps us survive. The theory is broken into three different states of our nervous system: social engagement, fight-or-flight, and freeze. These systems are evolutionary processes to support our survival.

> The foundational are functionally hardwired via "neuroception". Thus, although cues of safety or threat will trigger top-down reflexive changes in autonomic state, the states become associated with thoughts and behaviors. This process is initiated through interception and then bottom-up feelings of autonomic state are interpreted by higher brain structures, which in turn may initiate intentional behaviors. This linkage between feelings (i.e., autonomic state) and behaviors and thoughts form the neurophysiological basis for aspects of associative learning.
>
> (Porges, 2022, p. 4)

Porges identifies that the focus of many therapeutic strategies is to separate the feelings from the associative thoughts and behaviors. Therapeutic strategies that are "polyvagal-informed" focus on the experiencing of the feelings without linking to thoughts or behaviors (Dana, 2018; Porges & Dana, 2018).

This insight informs us, the provider or parent, to accept behaviors and feelings as adaptive responses that are important for the child (within their nervous system response) as a means of survival and not to stop the child or place shame for expressing these emotions. Then the child can be supported to anticipate the experiences (how feelings are felt in the body) and the expressed reactivity (the way in which the child protects him/her/their self) and then prevent the more nonpreferred responses (such as knowing how to physically slow down the body and breathe). Alternatively, the child can accept the current situation and inherent feelings and have a vast range of alternative coping responses.

In dance/movement therapy, I recognize the gut brain connection. The inherent locked state of fear response (adaptive survival responses) and the lack of habituation to the experience (for instance, the child responding as if this is the first time hearing a loud noise). I identify this state as the child's dial being turned up high (perceiving the environment or relationship to others with a heightened response or protected state). We look not to turn off the dial but rather to lower its intensity in an adequate response to the situation at hand as drawn in Figure 2.1.

Turning the dial

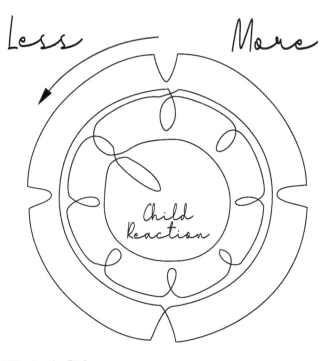

Less   More

Child
Reaction

Figure 2.1 Turning the Dial

Furthermore, it is essential to examine the modulation and balance of regulation – the process of achieving internal organization within the body through interactions with both the internal and external environment, including various experiences within different contexts (individuals, locations, objects). The bottom-up approach supports monitoring body sensations and resetting the nervous system.

The Sensory Plan

One way to better support the nervous system in children is through an intentional, sensory-driven plan during interactions. By selecting a child's regulatory preferences and delivering set environments and responses that produce a continuum of sensory feedback, each child becomes his/her/their best self. Learning how the child plays, soothes, and reacts provides essential insight into the day's schedule. Typically, I find children have been sharing this information with us all along. A child who wakes up quietly and examines the surrounding space is given an intentional plan that starts with visual activities, transitions into tactile input/touch, and so on. But a child who wakes up making noise may seek auditory input such as sounds, music, audio book, and deep proprioceptive input (e.g., massage, physical movement) to organize their system in order to start the day (Karim & Mohammed, 2015). Similarly, a child may sustain regulation when given a sensory diet that starts with physical (proprioceptive) input to awaken the body, followed by auditory listening to activate deep connection for promoting attention and following directions, and then visual stimulation to support curiosity, engagement, and communication. Setting up the child with a well-balanced routine plus a flow that meets their individual needs supports continued regulation. Over time, the routine and flow can be varied, the options expanded, and the regulation integrated.

When a child exhibits increased anxiety, upset, and defiance, we look at these intervention options for supporting the whole child in mind, body, and spirit. Acknowledging the child's sensory preferences and sensorial and movement patterns, and providing interactions that enlist the different sensory feedback preferences in a preferred order (sensory diet), can lead to optimal outcomes for everyone involved. Based on the theory of sensory integration, the sensory diet provides the child with sensory experiences throughout the day to maintain a balance of calm and alert state to meet the expectations and demands of the environment (Ayres, 1972; Wilbarger & Wilbarger, 1991). Strategies like working with sensory preferences and creating schedules can be helpful for all children, regardless of their diagnosis, in reducing anxiety and promoting inner awareness and developmental preferences. They can help children to feel calmer and more relaxed, to better understand their own emotions, and to develop the skills they need to cope with anxiety and stress. Additionally, these strategies bring familiarity, organization, and a sense of ease within the child's daily routine, which may typically be experienced as challenging.

Clinical Integration of DMT for Anxiety

In dance/movement therapy sessions, problem-solving and co-regulation with the child invite their individual profile into the session and build a framework for security. You will find this theme of safety present in all the vignettes and clinical-focus areas, such as the individual profile of the child (sensory needs and routines), movement profile and preferences (Chapter 1, Vignette 9), learning style, overall developmental needs, and more. Fortunately, these areas become second nature within the embodied practices, and the lens offers seamless attunement to the individual child. The common practice of mindfulness or being aware and present in the body is an active process that is not meant to be postulated as a rigid rule or challenging technique; thus, embodying the practice and allowing the body to move invites the inherent rapprochement of returning to the self for rest, recovery, and most importantly, the security and regulated flow a child needs to be receptive to learning and relating to their own process and the world around them (Bockmann & Yu, 2023; Murphy, Donna, Kohut, et al., 2022).

In the vignette titled "The Turtle" (Chapter 1, Vignette 2), the technique called mirroring activates the mirror neurons, which helps develop and promote empathy, attachment, and bonding (Berrol, 2006). Dance/movement therapists begin with mirroring to establish relationships and create a sense of safety. In mirroring, the therapist matches the individual's feeling tone, movement patterns, and effort qualities (Laban & Ullmann, 1971). As expressed in the vignettes, a child's movement profile is made up of various effort qualities – the way in which the movement feels and is perceived in action by the child and by the provider/parent. For example, this can be timing (how a child moves quickly or slowly), the child's use of weight (heaviness or lightness), and the directionality of movement (directly, from one point to another, or indirectly). These efforts are observed in all children and hold valuable information to intervention options and connections. Depending on the child and the goals for the session, while mirroring, the provider may for example amplify the child's movements by making them larger (taking up more space in the room or increasing the timing to a quick pace), or they might minimize them by making them softer/slower (moving to one location/point in the room, isolating the action to one part of the body, changing the weight lightly lifting or slowing down). The provider might gently shift the movement's effort and quality to make a more meaningful connection and intentionality in the therapeutic session (Berrol, 2006).

Carl Jung believed that humans have both a conscious and unconscious awareness, formed by archetypes (Jung, 1969). Archetypes are representations of behavioral patterns, symbols, and signs that have been passed down through generations, expressed in stories, and witnessed in our thoughts and experiences. (Adamski, 2011). Jung also believed the archetypal themes/images are the same for all humans, regardless of race, gender, age, or culture.

A dance/movement therapy original contributor, Mary Starks Whitehouse created the authentic movement approach (also referred to as active imagination in movement), which dance/movement therapists use to dive into the psyche when working with individuals (Whitehouse, 1979; Whitehouse & Pallaro, 1999; Stromsted, 2009). It is similar to Jung's approaches in that both practitioners believe humans connect through archetypes/images. Yet dance/movement therapy uses archetypes/images in combination with authentic/natural movement to support the individual's physical, emotional, mental, and social well-being. By diving deeper into the unconscious on a physical level, there is potential for transformation (Stromsted, 2009).

In dance/movement therapy, movement is key to understanding behavior and pathology. Ultimately, having a vast range of movement abilities and states creates an integrated, flexible, adaptive, social, cognitive, and emotional being. Conversely, rigidity, one dimensionality, or a lack of range depicts pathology, disease, and illness. We see that behaviors exhibited by an anxious child fit within the far ends of the spectrum of chaos (movements with asynchrony and disconnection) or rigidity (stiffening, withholding, and tension). These qualities are not personal; merely, they communicate physically the child's adaptive response to survive and protect (we will revisit this again in Chapter 7, Figure 7.1 The Integration Scale).

In "Goodbye Anxiety," (Chapter 1, Vignette 9), we learned about Willa's anxiety-based behaviors and her experience in a dance/movement therapy session. Research on trichotillomania has identified that "the majority (of children, and ongoing into adulthood) reported tension before pulling and gratification/relief immediately after pulling" (Woods & Miltenberger, 2007). This embodied description reinforces the importance of using movement in the presence of anxiety-related illnesses, such as pulling out hair and eyebrows. Because the symptom expression occurs in the body, this intervention is a direct path into and through the severe actions presented. Dance/movement therapy explores planes of movement to provide a framework for movement (Loman & Sossin, 2016). The planes can be explained as physical space in which the body occupies during held (stationary) or active (moving) interactions: horizontal, vertical, and sagittally taking up space or moving. This will be discussed more in Chapter 3.

When a child avoids movement in the vertical plane (up and down motion) and simultaneously does not stand up for themselves (literally), as in Willa's case, (Chapter 1, Vignette 9) we see that communication and problem-solving skills are compromised. As witnessed in the vignette, the movement planes act as a parallel process of the psychological and emotional state of the child.

Dr. Samaritter and Dr. Payne (2013), two dance/movement therapy researchers, state that research on sociology of human interactions points to the influences of held experiences (such as discourse) and that these experiences and patterns contribute to interactions that impact our emotional systems. This research acknowledges an understanding for the brain/body connection and the importance of regulation. The body contains stress in all its systems, whether the nervous system or the digestive tract, stored in the muscles and throughout the body. Treatment plans must understand and support this (Shaw, Labott-Smith, Burg, et al., 2018).

Linking Meaning and Authenticity

Brené Brown, the world renowned author and research professor, dispels the cultural myth that vulnerability is weakness. Brown provides insight into living authentically and how to create meaningful life experiences. Her findings speak to the relationship between holding feelings at bay, appearing to look astute versus genuinely revealing true feelings, and by taking risks, experiencing uncertainty, and expressing emotions openly (Brown, 2012). Her work emulates the connection and the integrated nature in which emotions are expressed in the body. Here we, the provider/parent, look to support the vast range of movement options: The ability to be flexible, adaptable, and "vulnerable" to open up and fully invite emotional expression. This common contradiction of vulnerability as weakness has the same effect on children, as explored in the vignettes. Tight composure can inhibit the child's ability to connect with others and navigate new experiences. The experience of more freedom in the body through movement allows for that identified strength that comes with being vulnerable. Additionally, the space for therapeutic movement enables a stronger relational bond with the therapist and helps the child move toward a connection to their emotional past and, ultimately, recovery.

Research shows the vast range of effects that trauma can cause for a person. As Peter Levine explained in his book, *Trauma Through a Child's Eyes*,

> Vulnerability to trauma differs from person to person depending on a variety of factors, especially age and trauma history . . . Trauma resides in the nervous system . . . Trauma is physiological rather than psychological . . . We are wired for survival.
>
> (Levine & Kline, 2006, p. 4)

We know that these experiences happen and are held in the body. The physiological experience is felt in the body and is dependent on the state of threat or safety. When the child embodies a state of postural strength (standing tall, holding shoulders straight and open), affective ease (smiling, relaxed muscles), and calm breathing, the child further experiences and feels these responses, allowing for healing and a reduction of stress/anxiety. This is why the movement approach is so critical in interventions used to support anxious children.

When clinicians treat these patterns as a lens into psychological challenges, they understand a child's behavioral movement and emotional needs. Bartenieff and Lewis (1980) identify the interplay of movement, the body, and the mind's determination in how one perceives and interacts. In their book, they discuss that when a pattern develops, such as a rigid or one-dimensional movement stance (stiffened joints, tense posturing), the individual's health is compromised and exhibited across the mind, body, and soul. For instance, in mending a wounded leg, it is not enough to just move the limb, but the mindset too; the emotional adherence to this movement and the will to move begins the healing process (Bartenieff & Lewis, 1980).

In dance/movement therapy, a parallel process occurs in which a child's movement choices, posture, and facial affect reflect the child's emotional experiences and body sense (Berrol, 2006). The dance/movement therapy lens of recognizing and attuning to the body such as mirroring the movement choices, joining the child's movements with a similar feeling tone/quality of movement, allow for a sense of being seen/supported. Additionally, the experience integrates in the brain/body as the cementing of new pathways; mirror neurons firing to create new, positive impressions, self-compassion, and connection (McGarry & Russo, 2011). Additionally, this method amplifies mindfulness practices, fostering progressive patterns in the body and mind in a nonjudgmental and active place of healing and growth.

The beautiful dance of using the body's movement promotes a space to integrate one's awareness of the anxious state while spontaneously and intuitively embodying a sense of knowing and repair. Again, the child feels the experience in the body, and the transformation occurs before her/his/their eyes.

Gauging the Truth

In the therapeutic interactions in Chapter 1, I acknowledged the individual's adaptive response toward his/her/their environment and situation. The children in the vignettes learned how thoughts contributed to feeling safe or unsafe. Additionally, the child learned to recognize whether their so-called barometer or gauge of the stressor or threat was adaptive, helpful, or counterproductive.

I love the Walt Disney quote, "Worrying is a waste of our imagination." The concept allows for the right combination of imaginative ideas and flights of fancy while maintaining a healthy curiosity and boundary for keeping threats at bay. If you have worked with me, you'll hear my constant recasting of the word "anxiety." I reinforce for the child that their response is not a diagnosis but an old reaction pattern, effective when there are real threats but not when the experience is a "just-right challenge," which can be predictable and a learning opportunity.

In an article from the Center on the Developing Child at Harvard University, the authors write that children with "chronic and intense fearful experiences often lose the capacity to differentiate between threat and safety" (Fox & Shonkoff, 2012, p. 73). These experiences impair the child's ability to learn and interact with others because they frequently perceive threats in ordinary social circumstances, such as on the playground or in school. Consequently, inhibiting the child's learning ability often leads to severe anxiety disorders. Fox and Shonkoff indicate that children may also express fear in response to situations similar to those they initially experienced or to conditions akin to the context in which the original learning occurred.

We can recognize the impact of this learned experience from the child's body posture, movement patterns, and relationship to the perceived threat. Similarly, a child's historical sensory disorganization (feeling like the body is under attack from textures, sounds, and lights; an imbalance of neuroception) can feel like a constant threat. The body's preference to find congruence (seek sameness) and make sense of the child's normal state (i.e., "I feel threatened; therefore, life is threatening") can perpetuate the ongoing spiral of despair.

The Environmental Impact

It would be remiss not to also mention the environmental link to mental health challenges. Whether we are looking at neurotoxicity, mold, infection, inflammation, dietary contributors, climate changes, pollution, exposure to technology, or the overall increasing, excessive demands, our children are overwhelmed, and expectations are heightened (Song, 2024; Katiraei & Bultron, 2011). During intake and throughout the therapeutic interactions, providers and parents can ask questions, and provide education around the impact of the environment on the body and the child's mental health. As identified in the vignettes, what was experienced in the body was expressed outwardly by the child into his/her/their relationships and social environments (Harding, Pytte, Page, et al., 2020). I have recognized patterns in the child's movements such as frenetic energy (emulating similarities seen from technology use), stuck movement themes and patterns (similar to inflammation swelling in the body), or attacking/fighting qualities (internally experienced as infection or threat), which provide a framework for further exploration, treatment options, and a path through the child's challenges.

This discussion extends further to include the embodied concepts of neurobiology in dance/movement therapy, in which the positive effects of dance/movement therapy on connections are explored. Kalila Homann, a licensed professional counselor-supervisor (LPC-S) and board-certified dance/movement therapist (BC-DMT), explores the use of synchrony, attunement, and emotional connectedness through movement and language. "Moving together creates a powerful relational experience and often stimulates a deep subjective feeling of connection" (Homann, 2010, p. 18). Sharing the situational load can diffuse the threat, and the pattern of stress/anxiety is effectively shifted. Attunement is an essential component of the therapeutic relationship and is encompassed in dance/movement therapy through the back-and-forth motions between individuals. Such as the mother-child relationship, the mutual attunement felt during interactions is based on needs and responses but also the movement rhythm and qualities expressed (Loman, White, & French, 2021). This experience of attunement requires a process of kinesthetic identification. Muscular tensions in one person feel the same in the other. It is not necessary to duplicate the shape of the movement. Visual or touch attunement with a child or caregiver can lead to calming. The degree of tension exhibited by the child or adult can be matched and then adapted to less intense, more soothing patterns (Loman, 1998; Malchiodi, 2005).

Once more, we observe how therapeutic movement and a unique perspective on the body serve as a means to provide alternative and holistic assistance in adjusting ingrained patterns, reinforcing positive new interactions, and gradually releasing the anxiety-inducing responses stored within the body and the mind's thoughts. In "Is Halloween Scary or Sweet?" (Chapter 1, Vignette 6), the child shows stress in the body. But therapeutic support enables access to a preferred state of being, which is the desired and accepted outcome.

Attunement

Stress can impact the brain-body connection. When a child experiences stress, the brain releases hormones that can disrupt the connection between the brain and the body. This can make it difficult for the child to regulate their emotions and behavior (Digitale, 2020). For instance, emotional stressors and responses impact a child's ability to communicate, problem-solve, and use executive-functioning skills to their fullest potential. Ultimately, providers and parents are encouraged to support a child's ability to regulate (to stay calm/alert) to complete tasks and manage life events. Approaches like security priming, a technique involving preemptively experiencing an event or action, along with practicing body postures and balance – adopting specific poses and stances to offer feedback and embody a desired state – have consistently demonstrated their effectiveness in mitigating anxiety and stress (Gokce & Harma, 2018, p. 3; Rodgers, Glod, Connolly, & McConachie, 2012; Stins, Ledebt, Emck, et al., 2009; Cuddy, Caroline, Wilmuth, & Carney, 2012).

Additionally, the therapeutic aim to understand the events leading up to the stressor to support rather than to stop the child's adaptive response to cope during or after the stressor has occurred acknowledges the child's need to release the emotional charge in order to return to the regulated state (Kapp, Steward, Crane, et al., 2019). For example, when working with children displaying stimulatory behaviors like hand flapping, repetitive sounds, or movement sequences, the objective is to decrease these patterns by addressing the instances when the child first feels overwhelmed or stressed. The aim is to extend their repertoire of behaviors by presenting substitute choices and a wider array of movements that can be suitable for the specific setting (e.g., hand flapping might evolve into options like shaking, holding, and pressing hands together). This approach ultimately fosters the spread of skills across different environments, promoting overall adaptability and embracing these variations (Wigham, Rodgers, South, et al., 2015). In finding this distinction of the time and delivery of movement, we can support the moments prior to the movement release and not hinder the child's expressive need and intentions. Utilizing the mind/body approach in psychotherapy sessions, as illustrated across the snapshots of moving moments vignettes, the child can develop awareness of their emotions (as expressed through words) and their increased attunement to their bodily sensations. This progression enables them to transition toward a posture of empowerment, synchronization with timing (rhythm and flow), and an overall sense of ease and increased comfort.

Call to Action

As we finish this section on anxiety, I want to share a common finding and a call to action: While empathy is the goal for our parent/child/provider relationship, you, the parent, or the provider have permission to differentiate and become the barometer that instills rational responses and lessons for the child. I recommend this because one typical response to an anxious state is the child's move to hijack the situation by negotiation. Negotiation is a reasonable attempt to control and navigate the unknown and delay the less-predictable, less-preferred situation. Parents get bombarded with words and may indeed regard the action as a witty display of brilliant ideas and creativity, not worth redirection, therefore giving in to their child's thoughts. In any other situation, talking and debating is a beautiful place for learning; in this case, however, limits, boundaries, and consistency will reduce the stressed state in these moments. The roots of the word "negotiate" – *nec* (not) and *otium* (free time/leisure) (Collins English Dictionary, 2024) – help us realize that it is not about free time to debate the undebatable. The parent is encouraged to omit the negotiation talk during these important transition moments and strive for clear communication and follow-through. Vast research shows how setting boundaries and clear expectations reduces anxiety and sets up a child for empathic, receptive, and direct communicative connection (Morris & March, 2004).

In "Riding the Bumps" (Chapter 1, Vignette 4), words that contributed to misunderstanding and judgment were omitted in the process of modeling embodied techniques of the parent/child dynamic in their control battle. The visceral experience was connected through a co-regulatory process, thus allowing for ease and recovery.

In a study of social baseline theory, researchers investigated the idea that having quality social relationships connects to having a long, happy life.

The human brain *expects* access to relationships, described as interdependence, shared goals, and joint attention. The researchers state,

> At its simplest, social baseline theory suggests that proximity to social resources decreases the cost of climbing the literal and figurative hills we face because the brain construes *social* resources as *bioenergetic* resources, much like oxygen or glucose. Indeed, evidence suggests that hills literally appear less steep when standing next to a friend.
>
> (Coan & Sbarra, 2015, p. 2)

Pain

Pain is defined in the dictionary as "physical suffering or discomfort caused by illness or injury" (Collins English Dictionary, 2024). Pain can be further characterized by considering its intensity range and discerning whether it manifests as an emotional sensation or is distinctly localized within a specific physical area of the body. As we explore the prevalence of pain that children experience in their bodies, it is important to note how the variables and etiology of pain differ depending on the illness, disease, injury, or exposure. In addition, emotional pain can alter one's experience of physical pain as the child relates imagery, memories, and relationships to the felt sense in their body.

To best support recovery, it is essential to allow acceptance of the child's pain. The book, *Perception of Pain*, explores how pain is interpreted by our past experiences, expectations, and even our culture (beliefs, rituals, and practices) not just the place on the body that has a wound (Print, 1974). As presented throughout these moving moments, children are given space to feel empowered rather than attempting to distract them from their pain. A child learns that their pain is real, both from their experience and with the provider witnessing/observing it. When therapeutic or medical treatment aims to distract a child, this action does not alleviate the route of the pain, nor does it allow for learning or resilience. By enabling the child to experience a new relationship with their body cues, whether relief or discomfort, the brain can change. With this plasticity, learning continues over the course of life (Siegel & Bryson, 2015). Additionally, the child can focus on their various senses and movement choices, reaffirming their options for insight into how pain feels, how they can or want to move, and if they want to stay in that feeling state or make any changes.

A randomized controlled study found that the intervention of somatic experiencing, in addition to treatment, had a significant effect on the participants who suffered from post-traumatic stress disorder (PTSD) and the connection to chronic pain (in this study chronic lower back pain) (Andersen, Lahav, Ellegaard, & Manniche, 2017). Somatic experiencing is a trauma therapy developed by Dr. Peter Levine that focuses on the body and sensations experienced in the musculoskeletal regions (Levine, 2008). Levine's trauma therapy emulates the lens of dance/movement therapy, with a focus on the body/mind connection and how emotions are experienced as sensations held in the body and identified as chronic pain or illness (Payne, Levine, & Crane-Godreau, 2015). In the dance/movement therapy sessions, (such as in Chapter 1, Vignette 1), the child can explore how their felt experience has a color, shape, texture, and movement, which provides meaning and recognition to know the emotion as it presents in the body.

Studies have found that by somatizing a patient's experience, individuals achieve a moderate reduction in their disability, pain, and acceptance of painless catastrophe. This outcome reiterates the benefits of changing fear networks through embodied practices, not just through exposure to memories (DeFano, Leshmen, & Ben-Soussan, 2019). Historically, pain is exclusively rated based on intensity and location, with limited connection to the processes surrounding an individual's cognitive or emotional relationship to pain and the pain scale (Maté, 2022). A bigger emphasis needs to be placed on the importance of psychological assessments (Williams, 2013). As a clinician, I have seen patients respond to a pain scale based on the emotional content of their illness, family dynamics, the intensity of the sensory experiences in the room, or the relationship/rapport with the staff member asking the rating-scale questions. By understanding the critical impact of the vast range of reactions to the child's pain and his/her/their connection to the pain, we can provide accurate interventions and collaborative connections.

Clinical Integration of DMT for Pain

In "Boiling Beans" (Chapter 1, Vignette 1), the use of a movement metaphor based on a painful memory of the child's mother making beans illustrates a key element of my work in dance/movement therapy with children. Often, physical pain has an emotional element to it, and through somatic analogies of connection, we can shift from tight and bound to lose and flowing. Using the body to access and gain control over painful emotions is a powerful method of shifting pain into comfort. Furthermore, somatic, and body-based practices such as dance/movement therapy show the efficacy of these practices for supporting pain, anxiety, and the experiences of post-traumatic stress symptoms (as indicated with trauma recovery) (Payne, Levine, & Crane-Godreau, 2015).

Recent research connects chronic pain with insecure adult attachment styles that originated in their early childhood experiences with primary caregivers (Tortora, 2006). Again, mindfulness and other body-based practices such as dance/movement therapy are successful therapeutic interventions for PTSD or those with traumatic upbringings that have led to chronic pain (Tortora, 2006). Yet this is another reason to support children moving through life, to relieve insecurity, anxiety, and pain later in life.

When we explore the body's response to pain, we can quickly identify the adaptive way that posturing and movements express the child's relationship to his/her/their discomfort. The pain mentality functions like a shield protecting the body from additional harm; however, this shield may also present with spikes and thorns as the child becomes agitated, antagonistic, and reactive (i.e., shutting out others). After the provider or parent indicates the connection and parallel between the posturing and presentation of pain for the child, appropriate interventions can be offered. Often, the child communicates an inability to move due to fear about more pain or discomfort. This highlights a lack of skills to make subtle adjustments and transitions, which are essential for achieving a state of comfort and ease. For my part, I often use the analogy, and verbalize to the child or parents, of being protected by cushions, blankets, and hugs instead of armor and weapons (i.e., fists, throwing objects, or pushing/kicking). Having multiple options for protection and the chance to gain more insight can provide an immediate path for the child to transform pain into relief instead of the reaction of the child to shut out others. By identifying the body's nonverbal communication, I have access to the child's view, supporting his/her/their control and improving their abilities to manage their perceived, uncontrollable state of pain. The body's movements become distinct, relatable, and felt when the provider can narrate and name the specific actions and movements displayed by the child in the specific context of the feelings and situation being revealed in the session.

In "Is My Child Acting With Aggression?" (Chapter 1, Vignette 10), we explore the dynamic of emotional pain. Research on the sociology of human interactions points to the influences of held experiences such as discourse and how these held experiences and patterns contribute to interactions and influence our emotional systems (Samaritter & Payne, 2013). The body holds stress in all systems, whether the nervous system or the digestive tract, and is held in the muscles and throughout the body. Treatment must understand and support it all (Pfeiffer, Shaunessy-Dedrick, & Foley-Nicpon, 2018; Van Der Kolk, 2014). The vignette supports the provider and parent to acknowledge the patterns of what may look like aggression (the physiological responses of discourse or stress throughout the child's development) that benefit from the therapeutic lens to accept, understand, and transform.

In "Can You Hear the Body?" (Chapter 1, Vignette 11), the therapeutic interaction supports the understanding and effectiveness of somatization. When a connection is made to the felt sense of the emotional and psychological concepts, as each occurs within the body and through movement, the child feels not only validated but also has a way to make the visceral feeling in the body purposeful and controlled (i.e., known). This known state provides color and shape, and, most importantly, the movement of the felt pain or body experience allows for the shift from thought to embodied relief. Hospital patients are often administered a standardized scale to rate their pain levels; however, their responses must be considered for they may also be indicative of their sensory and emotional openness to the therapeutic or medical dynamic. For instance, a child rating their existing pain as an 8 out of 10 (1 = no pain to 10 = highest level) in front of ten doctors may have increased the number due to feeling anxiety related to the imposition of questioning and the visual, auditory, and overall sensorial experience in the room. A more precise representation of a state of pain is achieved through somatization, wherein the senses evoke the location of pain within the body and the realization of its link to psychological experiences (Ogden & Minton, 2000). For change to occur within the child's health and emotional regulation, a greater awareness must be placed on somatic connections within the body and during medical and developmental care.

One method within dance/movement therapy focuses on four main categories of movement: body, effort, space, and shape. Teaching these main categories effectively has been shown to support changes in movement patterns, as further explored in Laban Movement Analysis (Bales, 2006; Laban & Ullmann, 1971). Laban's theory of "space harmony" posits that moving in specific directions in space (the physical room we are occupying and/or the areas around our physical body) naturally aligns with specific efforts (movement dynamics components such as light, strong, sudden, sustained qualities) and shape components (changes in the body's configuration such as sinking, rising, spreading, retreating). For example, reaching upward (in space) often lengthens the torso, which takes one into rising and supports lightness. In contrast, downward flexion (in space) may shorten the torso with sinking and facilitates strength (Tsachor & Shafir, 2017, p. 5).

You can picture these movement elements within relational exchanges between child, provider, parent, and peers. Imagine if the body is expressing a "shrinking" posture when ultimately a "rising" pattern would be more indicative of the intentional exchange. For instance, a child communicating about having a positive day would be matched with an upright torso and their head held high. By observing movement postures and the synchronous or asynchronous relation to the child's verbal communication, the provider and parent then have immediate information about the reality and true felt experience of that child. Supporting the child to find symmetry between what is said and what is expressed can create new pathways in the brain (neuroplasticity) to be authentically clear and intentional both internally (feeling) and externally (expression).

Collaboration

Clinical research has found that child therapy can only be successful if there is significant change within the parents or family dynamic, and this dynamic is felt and seen in the body shape and movement qualities (Gvion & Bar, 2014). Providers can support parent and child to recognize one another's movement patterns and make strides to truly read the body of the child. Understanding the discovery of neuroplasticity and the malleability of the brain in childhood and throughout life brings added eminence to how we continue to foster healing and connected relationships.

> This snapshot of interpersonal neuroscience is the first layer of a system that builds to suggest how relationships with self and with others result in growth, producing integration of the thinking/feeling/remembering aspects of one's brain; an integration that moves us toward a healthy mind and meaningful life.
>
> (Delaney & Ferguson, 2014, p. 146)

In "Shedding Light on Comfort" (Chapter 1, Vignette 13), the visual-spatial connection made during the intervention demonstrates the clinical application of how relationship building takes place. The therapeutic space and, further, the space occupied by the child, sheds light on his/her/their connection to and need for control, decreased anxiety, and reduced pain. Additionally, as shared in the vignette, props bring an element of safety to the therapeutic connection and a visual structure for the child to observe and measure. The vast range of nuanced techniques used in dance/movement therapy allows for the embodied practices of cognitive and psychological states. "Recently, it has been suggested that more subtle processes related to the therapeutic relationship and embodied cognition may be common underlying mechanisms associated with emotion regulation and fear extinction across therapeutic approaches" (Andersen, Lahav, Ellegaard, & Manniche, 2017, p. 2).

Additionally, the collaborative experience allows for sharing the pain load to reduce stress and ultimately alleviate the pain state (Sturgeon & Zautra, 2016). The provider models for the parent and family how to join the child to alleviate the burden, while also understanding what is occurring when a child turns internal feelings outwardly onto a parent. The principles identified in science, philosophy, and even some religious practices speak to leaning into the unknown and one's identified pain, which enables change to occur. The practice of meditation invites a state of awareness (at times a less familiar and unknown way of being), sensing all feelings of the body, and accepting the feelings while practicing breathing, movement, and stillness to best understand and aide in pain reduction (Sollgruber, Bornemann-Cimenti, Szilagyi, & Sandner-Kiesling, 2018). Furthermore, when we have the child differentiate the areas of the body in which the pain is located and acknowledge the distinction between that area and the rest of the body's sense of ease (or felt relief) in comparison, the child may then explore options and begin to find meaning within their experiences. The differentiation between being in pain (I feel pain therefore I exist as a child only in pain) and feeling pain in a specific area of the body (I have pain in my leg) and now the whole body provides feedback and further insight for supporting the child.

Awareness

As mentioned, traditional methods look to distract from or avoid pain or disturbance, which may prolong isolative, unaware/unyielding states, and a lack of empathic attunement to the individual's needs or options for growth and change. In the *Journal of Pediatric Nursing*, Koller and Goldman (2012) create a critical review of the literature expanding on the range of types of distraction techniques and support reasons for acknowledging individual child differences and child awareness for best practices. The therapeutic alliance through the mind/body connection provides permission to acquire a known state of awareness, through the body, imagery, and movement. Again, an understanding of and recognition of the full body state, differentiated areas of the body, and the existence of multiple ways of feeling at one time (i.e., I have pain in my leg but also a feeling of ease in my head, and even happiness in my heart). The child's individual experience, perceptions, feelings, and choices are given validity.

Within the therapeutic setting it's important to find curiosity and an ability to stay in the present moment, a common theme established in Eastern medicine that has provided endless support for those in need across history. The child can feel and be met in a shared experience of their rich emotional state, amid all the information it provides. For example, I have witnessed a child find comfort when we identified that his pain was in one area of his leg. Rather than trying to avoid the pain and focus on listening to a podcast, we decided together to listen to what we could imagine his leg was saying. The child communicated that *the leg* was not talking, but rather was screaming and shouting out. The child proceeded to communicate about the infections and then the surgeries the leg had been going through and how he had a voice now to speak up. Collaboratively, the child and I could hold space for a conversation, an opportunity for repair. To expand further, this child (like many others) didn't openly verbalize feelings to his parents and doctors, and so the benefit of having his leg speak out was a useful and effective outlet for self-reflection and communication.

Identifying the messages revealed through pain brings strength and insight to our human experience. Though pain is often met by an action to dispel or relieve, pain in the space of acceptance is viewed as a movement toward information, change, and healing. The therapeutic interaction between child and family members to accept the pain state, not of course to wish this on them or prolong it, but rather to ameliorate the associated fear and avoidance of this incredible state of information felt in the body. While child development may teach how to name feelings, in my therapeutic exchanges, I focus on the accuracy of what is felt and seen through movement, opening the possibility that what we feel is more than just one thing. A child feels pain in one area while also feeling an absence of pain in another area. A child feels fear, relief, love, exhaustion, comfort, and curiosity. The body shifts and tenses, releases, and moves, all with the experience of pain in conjunction with other states and expressions. With this understanding, movement becomes the truest form of dance for health and connection.

References

Adamski, A. G. (2011). Archetypes and collective unconscious compared to development quantum psychology. *Neuro Quantology: An Interdisciplinary Journal of Neuroscience and Quantum Physics*, 9(3). https://doi.org/10.14704/nq.2011.9.3.413

Andersen, T. E., Lahav, Y., Ellegaard, H., & Manniche, C. (2017). A randomized controlled trial of brief somatic experiencing for chronic low back pain and comorbid post-traumatic stress disorder symptoms. *European Journal of Psychotraumatology*, 8(1), 1331108.

Ayres, J. (1972). *Sensory integration and learning disabilities*. Western Psychological Services.

Ayres, J., & Robbins, J. (2005). *Sensory integration and the child: Understanding hidden sensory challenges*. Western Psychological Services.

Bales, M. (2006). Body, effort, and space: A framework for use in teaching. *Journal of Dance Education*, 6(3), 72–77. https://doi.org/10.1080/15290824.2006.10387318

Bartenieff, I., & Lewis, D. (1980). *Body movement: Coping with the environment*. Psychology Press.

Berrol, C. F. (2006). Neuroscience meets dance/movement therapy: Mirror neurons, the therapeutic process and empathy. *The Arts in Psychotherapy*, 33(4), 302–315.

Bockmann, J. O., & Yu, S. Y. (2023). Using mindfulness-based interventions to support self-regulation in young children: A review of the literature. *Early Child Educ Journal*, 51(4), 693–703.

Brown, B. (2012). *Daring greatly: How the courage to be vulnerable transforms the way we live, love, parent and lead*. Bren Brown. Gotham Books.

Carabotti, M., Scirocco, A., Maselli, M. A., & Severi, C. (2015). The gut-brain axis: Interactions between microbiota, central and enteric nervous systems. *Annals of Gastroenterology*, 28(2), 203–209.

Cisler, J. M. (2017). Childhood trauma and functional connectivity between amygdala and medial prefrontal cortex: A dynamic functional connectivity and large-scale network perspective. *Frontiers in Systems Neuroscience*, 11, 29. https://doi.org/10.3389/fnsys.2017.00029

Coan, J. A., & Sbarra, D. A. (2015). Social baseline theory: The social regulation of risk and effort. *Current Opinion in Psychology*, 1, 87–91. https://doi.org/10.1016/j.copsyc.2014.12.021. www.treatmentplansthatworked.com/EPSDT%20documents/CDC-ICDL%20Collaboration%20Report.pdf

Collins English Dictionary. (2024). Retrieved January, 2024. www.collinsdictionary.com/english/negotiate

Cuddy, A., Caroline, J. C., Wilmuth, A., & Carney, D. R. (2012). *The benefit of power posing before a high-stakes social evaluation*. Harvard Business School Working Paper, No. 13–027, September.

Dana, D. (2018). *The polyvagal theory in therapy: Engaging the rhythm of regulation* (Norton Series on Interpersonal Neurobiology). W. W. Norton & Company.

DeFano, A., Leshem, R., & Ben-Soussan, T. D. (2019). Creating an internal environment of cognitive and psycho-emotional well-being through an external movement-based environment: An overview of quadrato motor training. *International Journal of Environmental Research and Public Health*, 16, 1–20. https://doi.org/10.3390/ijerph16122160

Delaney, K. R., & Ferguson, J. (2014). Peplau and the brain: Why interpersonal neuroscience provides a useful language for the relationship process. *Journal of Nursing Education and Practice*, 4(8), 145.

Diamond, A. (2016). Why improving and assessing executive functions early in life is critical. In J. A. Griffin, P. McCardle, & L. S. Freund (Eds.), *Executive function in preschool-age children: Integrating measurement, neurodevelopment, and translational research*. The American Psychological Association.

Dictionary. (2023). *Wikipedia*. https://en.wikipedia.org/wiki/Dictionary.com

Digitale, E. (2020). *Stanford study finds stronger one-way fear signals in brains of anxious kids*. Stanford Medicine.

Farran, C. J., Miller, B. H., Kaufman, J. E., & Davis, L. (1997). Race, finding meaning, and caregiver distress. *Journal of Aging and Health*, 9(3), 316–333.

Fox, N. A., & Shonkoff, J. P. (2012). How persistent fear and anxiety can affect young children's learning, behaviour and health. In *Social and economic costs of violence: Workshop summary* (p. 69). National Academies Press.

Gokce, A., & Harma, M. (2018). Attachment anxiety benefits from security priming: Evidence from working memory performance. *PLoS One*, 13(3), e0193645. https://doi.org/10.1371/journal.pone.0193645

Gvion, Y., & Bar, N. (2014). Sliding doors: Some reflections on the parent–child–therapist triangle in parent work–child psychotherapy. *Journal of Child Psychotherapy*, 40(1), 58–72.

Harding, C. F., Pytte, C. L., Page, K. G., Ryberg, K. J., Normand, E., Remigio, G. J., DeStefano, R. A., Morris, D. B., Voronina, J., Lopez, A., Stalbow, L. A., Williams, E. P., & Abreu, N. (2020). Mold inhalation causes innate immune activation, neural, cognitive and emotional dysfunction. *Brain, Behavior, and Immunity*, 87, 218–228.

Homann, K. B. (2010). Embodied concepts of neurobiology in dance/movement therapy practice. *American Journal of Dance Therapy*, 32(2), 80–99.

Jung, C. G. (1969). *The archetypes and the collective unconscious*. Princeton University Press.

Kapp, S., Steward, R., Crane, L., Elliott, D., Elphick, C., Pellicano, E., & Russell, G. (2019). People should be allowed to do what they like: Autistic adults' views and experiences of stimming. *Autism*, 23(7), 1782–1792. https://doi.org/10.1177/1362361319829628

Karim, A. E., & Mohammed, A. H. (2015). Effectiveness of sensory integration program in motor skills in children with autism. *Egyptian Journal of Medical Human Genetics*, 16(4), 375–380.

Katiraei, P., & Bultron, G. (2011). Need for a comprehensive medical approach to the neuro-immuno-gastroenterology of irritable bowel syndrome. *World Journal of Gastroenterology*, 17(23), 2791–2800.

Kolacz, J., Kovacic, K. K., & Porges, S. W. (2019). Traumatic stress and the autonomic brain-gut connection in development: Polyvagal theory as an integrative framework for psychosocial and gastrointestinal pathology. *Developmental Psychobiology*, 61(5), 796–809.

Koller, D., & Goldman, R. D. (2012). Distraction techniques for children undergoing procedures: A critical review of pediatric research. *Journal of Pediatric Nursing*, 27(6).

Laban, R., & Ullmann, L. (1971). *The mastery of movement*. https://eric.ed.gov/?id=ED059225

Lebrun-Harris, L. A., Ghandour, R. M., Kogan, M. D., & Warren, M. D. (2022). Five-year trends in US children's health and well-being, 2016–2020. *JAMA Pediatrics*, 176(7), e220056.

Levine, P. A. (2008). *Healing trauma: A pioneering program for restoring the wisdom of your body.* Sounds True, Inc.

Levine, P. A., & Kline, M. (2006). *Trauma through a child's eyes: Awakening the ordinary miracle of healing.* North Atlantic Books.

Loman, S. (1998). Employing a developmental model. *American Journal of Dance Therapy,* 20(2), 101–115.

Loman, S., & Sossin, M. K. (2016). The Kestenberg movement profile in dance/movement therapy: An introduction. In *The art and science of dance/movement therapy: Life is dance* (2nd Ed., Vol. 2, pp. 255–284). Routledge/Taylor & Francis Group.

Loman, S., White, H., & French, M. J. (2021). Kestenberg Movement Profile (KMP) approaches to working with young children and caregivers in dance/movement therapy. *Journal of Infant, Child, and Adolescent Psychotherapy: JICAP,* 20(1), 36–50.

Malchiodi, C. A. (2005). Art therapy. In C. A. Malchiodi (Ed.), *Expressive therapies* (Vol. 220, pp. 16–45, xx). Guilford Press.

Maté, G. (2022). *The myth of normal: Trauma, illness, and healing in a toxic culture.* Penguin Publisher.

McGarry, L. M., & Russo, F. A. (2011). Mirroring in dance/movement therapy: Potential mechanisms behind empathy enhancement. *The Arts in Psychotherapy,* 38(3), 178–184.

Morris, T. L., & March, J. (2004). *Anxiety disorders in children and adolescents.* Guilford Press.

Murphy, S., Donna, A. J., Kohut, S. A., Weisbaum, E., Chan, J. H., Plenert, E., & Tomlinson, D. (2022). Mindfulness practices for children and adolescents receiving cancer therapies. *Journal of Pediatric Hematology Oncology Nursing,* 39(1), 40–48.

Ogden, P., & Minton, K. (2000). Sensorimotor psychotherapy: One method for processing traumatic memory. *Traumatology,* 6(3), 149–173. https://doi.org/10.1177/153476560000600302

Park, A. T., Leonard, J. A., Saxler, P., Cyr, A. B., Gabrielli, J. D. E., & Mackey, A. P. (2018). Amygdala-medial prefrontal connectivity relates to stress and mental health in early childhood. *Social Cognitive and Affective Neuroscience,* 13, 430–439. https://doi.org/10.1093/scan/nsy017

Payne, P., Levine, P. A., & Crane-Godreau, M. A. (2015). Somatic experiencing: Using interoception and proprioception as core elements of trauma therapy. *Frontiers in Psychology,* 6, 93.

Pfeiffer, S. I., Shaunessy-Dedrick, E., & Foley-Nicpon, M. (2018). *APA handbook of giftedness and talent.* American Psychological Association.

Porges, S. W. (2022). Polyvagal theory: A science of safety. *Frontiers Integrative Neuroscience,* 16.

Porges, S. W., & Dana, D. (2018). *Clinical applications of the polyvagal theory: The emergence of polyvagal-informed therapies* (Norton Series on Interpersonal Neurobiology). W. W. Norton & Company.

Print, O. O. (1974). *Puz of pain.* Basic Books.

Rodgers, J., Glod, M., Connolly, B., & McConachie, H. (2012). The relationship between anxiety and repetitive behaviours in autism spectrum disorder. *Journal of Autism and Developmental Disorders,* 42(11), 2404–2409. https://doi.org/10.1007/s10803-012-1531-y

Rolls, E. T. (1992). Neurophysiology and functions of the primate amygdala. In J. P. Aggleton (Ed.), *The amygdala: Neurobiological aspects of emotion, memory, and mental dysfunction* (Vol. 615, pp. 143–165, xxi). Wiley-Liss.

Samaritter, R., & Payne, H. (2013). Kinaesthetic intersubjectivity: A dance informed contribution to self-other relatedness and shared experience in non-verbal psychotherapy with an example from autism. *The Arts in Psychotherapy,* 40(1), 143–150.

Schulkin, J., McEwen, B. S., & Gold, P. W. (1994). Allostasis, amygdala, and anticipatory angst. *Neuroscience and Biobehavioral Reviews*, 18(3), 385–396.

Shaw, W., Labott-Smith, S., Burg, M., Hostinar, C., & Alen, N. (2018). *Stress effects on the body*. Am Psychol Assoc.

Siegel, D. J., & Bryson, T. P. (2015). *No-drama discipline: The whole-brain way to calm the chaos and nurture your child's developing mind*. Scribe Publications.

Sollgruber, A., Bornemann-Cimenti, H., Szilagyi, I.-S., & Sandner-Kiesling, A. (2018). Spirituality in pain medicine: A randomized experiment of pain perception, heart rate and religious spiritual well-being by using a single session meditation methodology. *PLoS One*, 13(9), e0203336. https://doi.org/10.1371/journal.pone.0203336

Song, E. (2024). *Healthy kids, happy kids: An integrative pediatrician's guide to whole child wellness*. Harper Collins Publishers.

Stins, J. F., Ledebt, A., Emck, C., Van Dokkum, E. H., & Beek, P. J. (2009). Patterns of postural sway in high anxious children. *Behavioral and Brain Functions*, 5, 42. https://doi.org/10.1186/1744-9081-5-42

Stromsted, T. (2009). Authentic movement: A dance with the divine. *Body, Movement and Dance in Psychotherapy*, 4(3), 201–213. https://doi.org/10.1080/17432970902913942

Sturgeon, J. A., & Zautra, A. J. (2016). Social pain and physical pain: Shared paths to resilience. *Pain Management*, 6(1), 63–74.

Taylor, A. G., Goehler, L. E., Galper, D. I., Innes, K. E., & Bourguignon, C. (2010). Top-down and bottom-up mechanisms in mind-body medicine: Development of an integrative framework for psychophysiological research. *National Library of Medicine*, 6(1), 29–41.

Tortora, S. (2006). *The dancing dialogue: Using the communicative power of movement with young children*. Paul H. Brookes Pub.

Tsachor, R. P., & Shafir, T. (2017). A somatic movement approach to fostering emotional resiliency through Laban movement analysis. *Frontiers in Human Neuroscience*, 11, 410.

Van Der Kolk, B. A. (2014). *The body keeps the score: Brain, mind, and body in the healing of trauma*. Penguin Books.

Whitehouse, M. S. (1979). C.G. Jung and dance therapy: Two major principles in eight theoretical approaches in dance-movement therapy. In P. L. Bernstein (Ed.), *Eight theoretical approaches in dance movement therapy*. Kendall/Hunt.

Whitehouse, M. S., & Pallaro, P. (1999). *Authentic movement: Moving the body, moving the self, being moved: A collection of essays* (Vol. 2). Jessica Kingsley Publishers.

Wigham, S., Rodgers, J., South, M., McConachie, H., & Freeston, M. (2015). The interplay between sensory processing abnormalities, intolerance of uncertainty, anxiety and restricted and repetitive behaviours in autism spectrum disorder. *Journal of Autism and Developmental Disorders*, 45(4), 943–952. https://doi.org/10.1007/s10803-014-2248-x

Wilbarger, P., & Wilbarger, J. (1991). *Sensory defensiveness in children ages 1–12: An intervention guide for parents and other caretakers*. Avanti Educational Programs.

Williams, D. A. (2013). The importance of psychological assessment in chronic pain. *Current Opinion in Urology*, 23(6), 554–559.

Woods, D., & Miltenberger, R. (2007). *Tic disorders, trichotillomania, and other repetitive behavior disorders: Behavioral approaches to analysis and treatment*. Springer Science & Business Media.

Chapter 3

The Therapeutic Lens Explored

Critical Areas in Children – Neurodivergence and Asynchronicity

When I started working with children diagnosed on the autism spectrum, I was immediately amazed by the differences in each child's early life experiences, medical needs, and learning styles. I recall being asked countless questions by parents who wondered whether the autism spectrum disorder (ASD) diagnosis could be "fixed" or "go away." Since that is a loaded question with much variability, I responded by asking, "What are you hoping your child or family members can achieve/experience?" Armed with the information their answers provided, we found important, creative, and whole-body interventions to support growth and development. Through dance/movement therapy, a child who presents with neurodivergence (neurological variations in sensory processing, emotional/developmental/physical challenges, and asynchronistic cognitive learning differences) can start to be understood and accepted into the family home and social world. Our supportive strategies can follow suit when we are clear in what we are asking.

I am aware of the sensitivity of exploring this topic and the emotional vulnerability and strength that family members and loved ones manage as they work to support the neurodiverse child or one with an ASD diagnosis. This analysis brings further awareness to how we can collectively provide understanding and acceptance of the paths leading to symptoms while continuing to promote health and growth.

Diagnosis Expanded

The concept of a diagnosis was created to allow for clarification among professionals and ease in describing symptoms with consistency. For example, rather than telling a colleague about a client with social impairment, nonverbal communication deficits, and lack of eye contact (to name a few), the provider could say ASD. However, when resorting to diagnostic labels, there's a risk of losing the nuances of symptoms and, more importantly, the core of each child's unique experience. This can give rise to stigmas and unfounded assumptions. The diagnosis does not look at

DOI: 10.4324/9781003363491-4

etiology, the why of how symptoms develop in the first place, nor the adaptive nature of the child's ability to respond to the world in order to protect and guard for survival. Understanding how a child comes to present symptoms – or movements, as I call them – and the nature/nurture of that child greatly supports our therapeutic role within the family system, the treatment methods, and the additional lens through which we serve the child and family.

If we look at the ASD population, specific symptoms associated with ASD, and its widespread numbers, we can also see varying degrees of etiology. I can decipher five different areas of explanation:

1. The child who presents with autistic symptomatology without the following additional impairments or challenges.
2. The child who had early life trauma such as but not limited to loss, acculturation, abuse, and neglect.
3. The child with early medical needs such as seizure disorders, physical impairments/illness, otitis media, or mold toxicity/autoimmune dysfunctions.
4. The child may have learning differences such as dyslexia, asynchronous/gifted/2e, or sensory deficits and comorbid disorders like obsessive-compulsive disorder and attention deficit disorder.
5. The child with diagnosed personality disorders, reactive attachment, psychological disruption/imbalance, and diagnostic indication.

The point of these distinctions is not to place blame on anyone or any specific event or environment to determine "who it came from," or to upset those that rely on a diagnosis. Rather, I am making these distinctions to develop best practices and a wider lens through which to view and support the foundation of the individual and whole child. I find that these children all fit the criteria and are given the diagnosis of ASD because the symptoms present in a consistent manner, and this is specifically why the providers and parents need to discern etiological factors to best apply intervention practices, family support, and individualized approaches that look at the whole child.

Many experts in child development discuss the foundation and underlying components of the child to support optimal health (Delahooke, 2019; Birkland, 2007). The foundation (those bottom-up aspects of the child); physiological states, including neuroception, emotional and stress responses, and sensory processing, (that impact the child's presentation or behaviors) is a critical place to acknowledge and further support neurodivergent children. By looking at the individualized profiles of a child presenting with similar symptoms and then expanding past the criteria of ASD into the vast areas of treatment, the family can have a clear understanding of support for their child and options for care.

Therapeutic Lens

Through the dance/movement therapy lens, I consider neurodivergence to be another embodied manifestation of individual differences. The asynchronous body movements and patterns are seen physically and expressively displayed in a child, known as 2e, or twice exceptional (Arky, 2023). The visual appearance of the body movements, patterns, and asynchronous postures of the asynchronous child – this parallel presentation – and the connection to the child's mental, social, and physical experiences, states, and needs provide added information for clinical care. There is an ebb and flow of changes that occur throughout a given interaction. Whether a five-year-old child presents like an adult scientist, a toddler in tantrum mode, or a teen sports fanatic, the body movements, posture, and facial affect switch while the physical identity of the child may seem the same. Again, when we look at the body, we can parent and support the child in front of us without comparison or judgment: The held-together arms of the little scientist, ready to collapse if his experiment fails; the tantrummer's tense body posture and tilted head; the sports fanatic who moves seamlessly during the sport but falters when slowing down (not unlike the spinning top that appears so deft when in constant motion but immediately starts to wobble when slowed down).

By looking at the body, the provider and parent can identify what is to come while staying focused on the present expression in front of them. When a disparity in skills is evident – such as a child being academically advanced but demonstrating social, emotional, or regulatory abilities akin to a younger age – this incongruity manifests in an array of assorted behaviors. When a child presents consistently on varied skills (even highly achieving across skill levels or relatively standard across levels), we see minimal challenges. The disparity is the key to which the child may know what and how to be while presenting otherwise, or vice versa. Here we work to find a balance between the areas and to provide more consistency for the child across skills. We may celebrate strengths while acknowledging the significant discrepancy between one skill and another.

This distinction places importance on supporting a child physically and psychologically through developmental milestones. Stanley Greenspan's and Serena Weider's floor time model, a kindred lens to my dance/movement therapy modality brings focus to the embodied process of moving a child from regulation to joint attention, communication, and problem-solving, all leading to more critical thinking, abstract thought, and inner contemplation. The child physically moves up the developmental ladder and returns down, repeating patterns and solidifying pathways for learning and integration (Wieder & Greenspan, 2003; Greenspan & Wieder, 2007; Cordero, Greenspan, Bauman, et al., 2006). The impact of relationships on well-being is further validated in therapeutic interventions like those used in the developmental, individual-differences, relationship based model (DIR). "As a functional approach, it uses the complex interactions between biology and experience to understand behavior and articulates the developmental capacities that provide the foundation for higher-order symbolic thinking and relating" (Wieder & Greenspan, 2003, p. 2).

During these therapeutic sessions, led by a therapist, a parent and child have access to affective tone, gestures, words, and movement support so the child can "climb up the symbolic ladder" (Wieder & Greenspan, 2003, pp. 3–10). The ladder represents the multiple stages of developmental learning. By continuing to integrate body-focused strategies for understanding relational patterns and social needs within the therapeutic exchange, we validate the importance of the whole child family system. We now have an embodied understanding for the physicality and lived adaptive use of all the symptoms presented in the body by the child and with us, the provider, and parents.

If a child has "holes" in developmental milestones, a therapist may see challenges in maintaining these higher levels across environments and dynamics. A child may demonstrate problem-solving skills while needing support to communicate effectively with peers. Learning about the individual child's functional and emotional development, looking further at the parallels between these stages and the child's body movements holds significant value in supporting the child's developmental needs with supportive intervention. The therapist can access information through body movements displayed in sessions to know which interventions to provide, how to communicate to find meaningful connections, and to further support parents/providers in learning the patterns for ongoing growth and acceptance.

The therapist co-regulates with the child so that they can figuratively climb back through the functional emotional developmental levels and ultimately begin to regulate. Even in reading the various stages, we can see the embodied approach of integrating skills and movement-based relating (Mavilidi, Pesce, Benzing, et al., 2022).

Subtitles

With a child in these polarities, I look at what I call subtitles (see Figure 3.1): The feeling state under the child's words that reveals the child's internal process and congruence to his/her/their body state. Especially with asynchronous patterns, a child's words must be considered only while also observing the child's body language, stance, and body knowledge. A child who says no during a physical exchange, like transitioning, may indicate a need for more time, communicating that the transition was not their idea or that what they are doing is more important now. The subtitles provide a clue into the child's underlying intention and invite the observer to look at and listen to the body and not just the words.

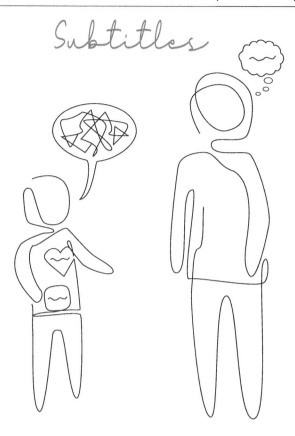

Figure 3.1 Subtitles

We may miss the authentic experience and feeling state when words take over our understanding. Consider the dialect, language, and words you know; but what is underneath, the actual English (or your native language), the subtitles, if you will, translate what feelings are present in the dynamic. I have a video of my daughter at three years old; in it, I asked her to sing a song, to which she replied, "No, no. . . ." But then she proceeded to sing the song after she finished eating. To read the "no" that is associated with "I won't do what you say" is not accurate here; the subtitles I read were, "Wait, I am finishing my food," after which she began to sing. I have supported parents' countless times to look past and under the words they hear to identify true feelings and needs. Listen to the body's phrasing, stance, and response posture. This method elicits a slowing down, creating accuracy between verbal and nonverbal communication. The goal is not to ignore our children's communication, but rather to ensure we identify what is accurate and valid for that moment.

Indeed, a child's vulnerability to their lower skill point (e.g., emotional regulation) leads them to defend and guard with their preferred strength, intellect, and words. The child may feel intensely and indicate a disparity between what is known and what is shown outwardly (i.e., knowledge in relation to or versus the child's emotional regulation or physical skill set), creating a discrepancy between the two levels. But when we invite the child to see how vulnerability can be a strength to share and learn from, acknowledging our awareness of their actual, subtitled language, we support their self-compassion and further connections. I like to call them "star children": Those from the galaxy, more ethereal and all-knowing, not one above the other or better than, but those in a space that transforms and changes daily. They are blessed with gifts – yes, gifts – that can cause challenges, misunderstandings, high expectations, and burnout. We must celebrate and acknowledge these children as they are and learn from them in our interactions.

When a child appears to lack empathy or presents with opposition, notice that empathy starts first with self-compassion. We must feel love for ourselves and know how to love intrinsically to share that love and support with others. When a child harms another, that child is feeling harmed too. When we look to the offender and not just the victim, we can support the meaningful connection of empathy. Realize that a child must be in their worst state, at their most vulnerable, to present with challenging, contrary behavior. If the child were feeling their best, the challenge would not occur. The child must not feel like a burden, bad, or belittled at that moment; rather, the child needs to be accepted, supported, and given a secure connection.

Concepts and Patterns

In my practice, I have noticed patterns forming around children's behaviors and what is accepted as appropriate. To honor a child's emotional states, mental and physical abilities, and environmental expectations, I think about frameworks that may help shape our adult responses. A younger child appears to have more room for behaviors of emotional dysregulation than an older child, for example. I have developed a concept called the principle of cuteness to help support parents and to inform my interns and colleagues about this precious work. In my principle of cuteness (see Figure 3.2), I acknowledge for parents that sometimes what a restless child does in their early years is seen as adorable, personally and culturally, but such behaviors quickly lose cuteness in the child's older years. Recognizing and responding to an anxious child invites opportunities for building resilience and space for absolute truths. So when a child responds through movement at a later age, seeing their behavior as not cute or unwelcome may cause more harm than help. Connection is the goal of cuteness, and

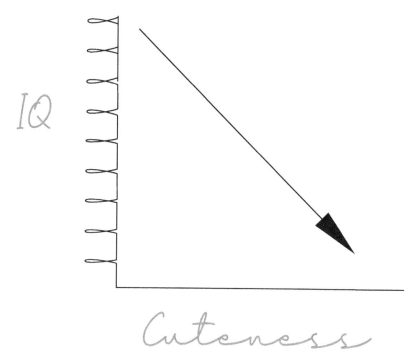

IQ

Cuteness

Figure 3.2 The Principle of Cuteness

that connection stays throughout life; the child needs and craves these types of interactions even at the most trying times.

Interestingly, while cuteness is a means to connect, often asynchronous kids with gifts and discrepancies leave the cuteness stage earlier, as soon as they can articulate their thoughts or physical skills are further developed. Society views *ability* as dominant, and the adorable baby/toddler is no longer present. Advanced skill sets generate heightened expectations for asynchronous children, which can further highlight their constrained capacity to sustain the connected and emotive states commonly experienced and expressed during the earlier years by neurotypical children. One example of an attempt to return to a younger stage of cuteness is displayed by the older child who regresses into using a baby voice, collapsed posture, or clings behind a parent. Historically, I've noted that feelings aren't immediately accepted when thoughts and intellect are allowed to take over the social exchange.

Because our systems are active, moving, and embodied, I'd like to postulate that when a child experiences internal processes, they must present congruent behaviors externally (actions presented in physical health and emotional expression). A child's body seeks congruence, an understanding that what feels true is valid. If the feeling and state are present, they must be relevant and accurate. Thus, the individual seeks this sameness in relationships with others and the environment. A child with internal dysregulation appears to be in a state of combativeness and the instigator of the fight. While fighting about transitions, with their parents' words and expectations, and the responses to their sensory world, the child isn't being "bad" or "difficult," but rather the child is looking for what is consistent and true. We can better understand, predict, and communicate our child's needs by supporting this outer movement as internal information (what we see outside becomes the window into what is internal). This is understood thoroughly in the gut-brain connection, our body's functional way of sending messages from the body to that brain, and our overarching theme for maintaining allostasis (balance state) (Maté, 2011).

For instance, in autoimmune disorders such as PANS or PANDAS (pediatric acute-onset neuropsychiatric syndrome/pediatric autoimmune neuropsychiatric disorder associated with streptococcal infections) a child harboring bodily toxicity might exhibit instances of flare-ups and outbursts characterized by toxic reactions within their environment (Gagliano, Carta, Tanca, & Sotgiu, 2023). In my practice and discussions with colleagues and families, we see these reactions all the time and consider the reports of the child having what appears like psychiatric symptoms of hearing voices or acting manic, as well as becoming physically destructive, and untamed at times while concurrently suffering internally from the toxicity of autoimmune challenges and inflammation (Silverman, Frankovich, Nguyen, et al., 2019).

Parallel Process

My observations of a child's movement indicate a parallel process to the internal orientation of the body (as present in disorders and diseases, alike). At pediatric hospitals, I have worked with chilren diagnosed with sickle cell disease, which I loosely describe as when the blood cells shape (due to the disorder) causes a blockage of the flow in distributing blood across the body. With this inflammation and blockage, the child experiences chronic and severe pain. What I find interesting and look forward to more research/perspectives on is that these children in sessions, utilizing dance/movement therapy, appear to have a flight of ideas, limited connection to sequencing, and a flow-to-stop rhythm. While, a child with autoimmune toxicity, a literal experience of the body attacking systems and working to rid mold and aversive allergic reactions, presents with outbursts. It is incredible to see the child's external relationships, presented content, and how they move creating a familiar pattern to their internal state. Making connections from internal disease to external patterns of movement supports reorganizing, reaffirming, and resolving the feeling states of pain and anxiety. Dance/movement therapy can support the child by matching their body's communication and seeing how that reflects their internal and external experience.

Bandwidth and Tolerance

A common theme in my clinical work is understanding the child's bandwidth and that of their family; appreciating each child's frustration tolerance and their tipping point, edge, or limitations supports the clinical work and focus for supportive treatment. Here, I use the metaphor of a pot of water (see Figure 3.3): We must understand that if we leave the lid on too tight, the water will flow out and bubble over, potentially evaporate, and the bottom of the pot will burn. Our job, therefore, is to make sure a little steam can escape from under the lid, sparingly and consistently, all

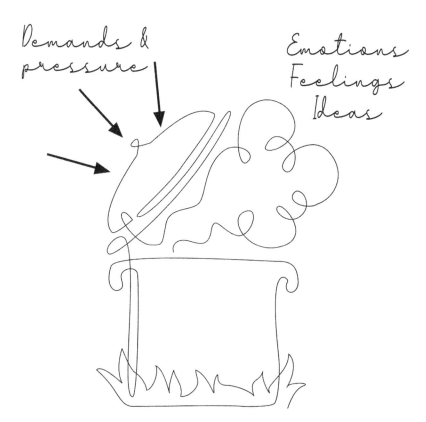

Figure 3.3 The Boiling Pot

while making that amazingly delicious, rich soup. A child's experiences are colored with people, objects, and environments, while emotions make up the ingredients and add the possibility of getting too hot (overspent). Focusing on the overload creates space for beautiful learning and enrichment without ruining the soup.

The emotional discord and outbursts we see in our children are not only indicative of upset, but they are also a release of feelings. I compare the expulsion or wringing out of the day's intensity to how a sponge releases water and dirt, ready to soak up suds and water again the next day (see Figure 3.4). Therefore, the release of big emotions is not evidence that something is wrong, per se, but rather it is a healthy wringing out of the day, offloading and rebooting, ready for what comes next.

Acceptance

I pride myself on supporting parents, providers, and even the child to experience the child's (their) behaviors (movements) and emotions as predictable

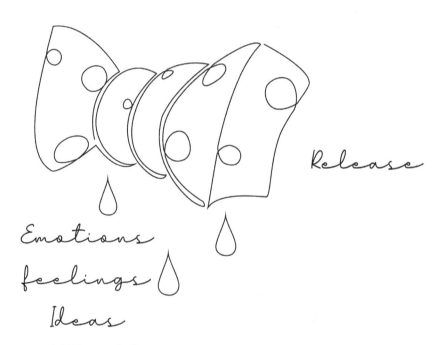

Figure 3.4 Wringing the Sponge

even when the situation or reaction may feel difficult to handle. Anticipating and knowing the predictability of the child's presented responses further supports parents in moving toward awareness and understanding of these differences rather than confusion. The questions shift from "Why are you doing that?" to "Oh, I knew that was likely, and now how can we be of support?"

I will continue offering my metaphors and analogies to viscerally, vividly, and tangibly relay scenarios we often cross in clinical work and to highlight the felt experience of the interventions.

When a parent leaves the playground but the child longs to stay, we cross paths with the child's resistance. These moments happen frequently, and the child's objection to completing the preferred task is considered a roadblock. Here, a hill metaphor (see Figure 3.5) can help the parent guide their child through the challenge: No matter what, we must climb the hill to get home, but our choice is in *how* we climb. A child can be made aware that leaving and accepting the action of moving through the moment of conflict will happen; the parent then proposes options for executing the moving part. Rather than relying on all-too-familiar, empathic, peaceful words about how the child feels, the parent must instead physically move through these moments. The child is presented with options for hopping, marching, piggyback riding, or skipping up the hill. Moving into the non-preferred transition, or leaving, becomes progressive and embodied. The challenge is no longer between the parent and child; it is now the hill, and the child and parent are a team.

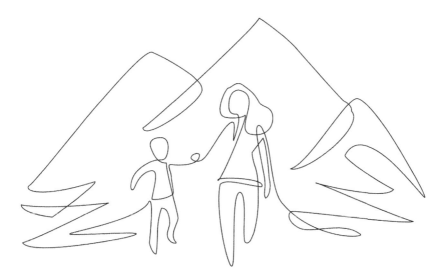

Figure 3.5 Climbing the Hill

Connection

For a child who is stuck and unable to work through the challenge, I use a rock-climbing metaphor (see Figure 3.6). When we look at the child in their challenged space, the problem is too far away. The child is isolated, panicked, and in a state of danger – say, at the top of a giant rock wall. If

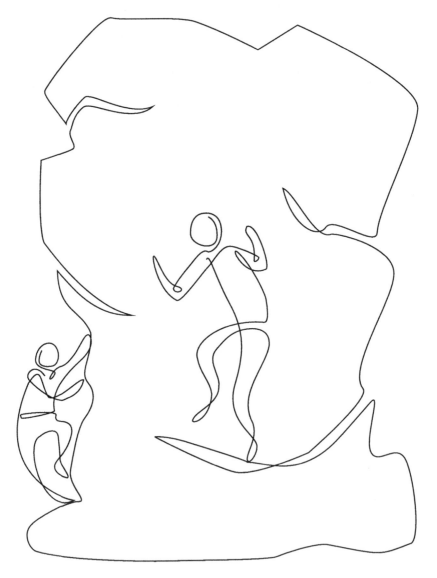

Figure 3.6 The Rock-Climbing Metaphor

we loudly call out to the child, the distress becomes too much as yelling intensifies the situation. Instead, we must physically reach their level, climbing up the wall to meet the child in that space, knowing where hands, legs, and feet land; what we can see; and what sounds are clear. Then the parent or provider can identify the next steps for moving down the rock wall, slowly and easily, back to solid ground. In real application, this concept works with a simple example of a child solving a complicated math assignment; in which yelling up to them to complete the work doesn't help, assuming the child can complete the math independently doesn't work, and yet, sitting next to them, breaking down the steps of the problem (using manipulatives to visually see the math on the table), and writing it together (moving your body collaboratively) supports the child to problem solve, become receptive to learn the skills, and ultimately complete the assignment. Most importantly, this ability to meet not in words but in a physical stance and body posture supports connections needed for sharing the stress load and embodying a healthy relationship. It's imperative in these moments to differentiate parent and child emotionally while linking physically – as the adult isn't being stuck in the hole or stranded on the mountain. The adult knows the way out mentally and has the wisdom to share, once and only when the two bodies are aligned, in sync, and connected in a trusting, safe manner. This important distinction promotes healthy body boundaries, internal awareness, and external reciprocity.

Benefits of DMT

Movement improves the human body's mental and physical well-being, including cardiovascular health, self-expression, self-confidence, and pure *joy*. The list of benefits may be endless. In a past collaboration with the American Heart Association and the American Dance Movement Foundation, activities that involved movement and dance were used to increase health, reaching more than *37,000 schools and 19 million kids* (american-dancemovement.org/health-initiative)! Movement is inside our bodies and laced through our interactions. We don't need to create it by physically jumping or dancing, per se; we need to acknowledge that we are always moving in life, through every heartbeat, breath, posture, and more.

Across many studies, social skills like smiling and verbalization are substantially higher when neurodiverse children engage in socially embedded motion versus sedentary activities like board games (Rafiei Milajerdi, Sheikh, Najafabadi, et al., 2021). Research indicates that movement activities improve coordination and balance, promote ease of breathing, increase relaxation, and decrease anxiety (Najafabadi, Sheikh, Hemayattalab, et al., 2018). Children may find novelty in technology and interactive programs, but they tire more of the sameness of such interactions compared with

Body

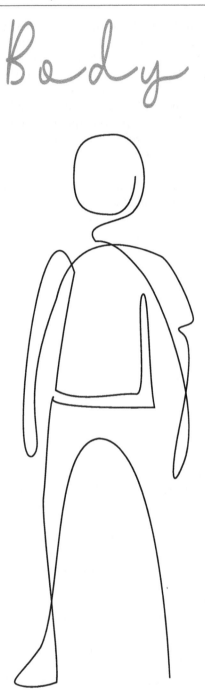

Figure 3.7 Body

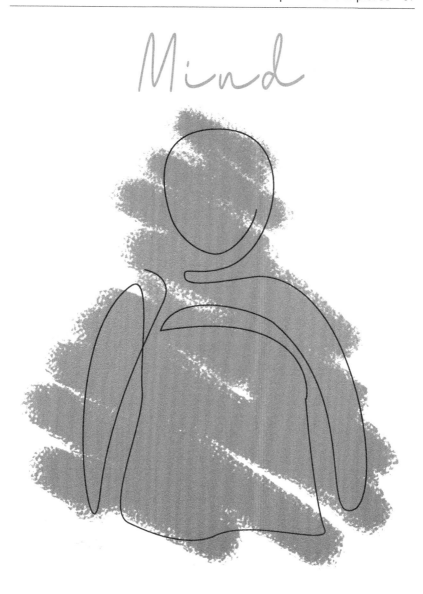

Figure 3.8 Mind

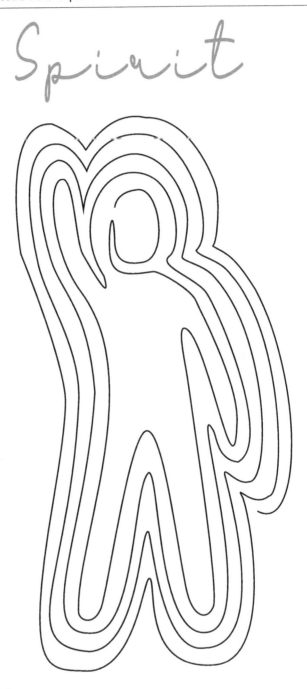

Figure 3.9 Spirit

dance, turn-taking, facial expressions, and naturally occurring dynamics. Thus, human contact promotes more compassion and excitement than mere skill. I recommend that what is done or viewed on a screen be embodied and expressed physically.

When we move through the dance of life, we generate more activity, repetition, and access as the mirror neurons fire; the specific neurons in the brain that activate when a sensorimotor experience is repeatedly acted as well as when seen by the individual (i.e., the baby mirroring the facial expressions of a parent or a dancer learning movement just by watching a performance on stage) (Heyes, 2010). This then supports reciprocity and engagement to follow and learn. Just look at the person next to you, and you'll find a mirroring of connected bodies. Dancing improves brain function and boosts memory. Studies show that dancing improves cerebral health and spatial memory, one of the cognitive domains (Kattenstroth, Kalisch, Holt, et al., 2013). Studies also suggest that maintaining an active lifestyle into old age can preserve motor, cognitive, and perceptual abilities. These ideas are linked to neuroplasticity, the brain's ability to form new neural connections and to change and adapt (Voss, Thomas, Cisneros-Franco, & de Villers-Sidani, 2019). So let's start with the children, through the ongoing practice of movement that positively affects brain activity (see Figures 3.7, 3.8, and 3.9) – in mind, body, and spirit.

Movement Explored

The body-based approach shown in each of the moving moments vignettes in Chapter 1 explore the premise, I have found in dance/movement therapy, that total integration and health enable an individual to move in full range with all polarities and movement styles at optimal times, such as knowing when to move quickly out of harm's way or how to easily connect in a vulnerable interaction. The flexibility of movement, its vast expressiveness, and variation promote a healthy, integrated space for ideal wellness and learning. The sessions described in Chapter 1 demonstrate the use of effort qualities; space, weight, and time (as discussed in Chapter 2); how a child interacts with the self and another and amid the variables of daily events, expectations, and emotional regulation.

The techniques used in dance/movement therapy are comprehensive, providing a lens that integrates psychology with spontaneity, individualized treatment, and playful learning. For example, the dance/movement therapy approach of authentic movement, which explores a child's inner imagination and body-felt experiences, resonates with legendary psychiatrists/psychoanalysts including Carl Jung's use of archetypes and collective consciousness. Authentic movement focuses on the individual's ability to stay connected to what the body (muscles, bones, facia, nerves, veins, pulse) intends, not just what a person thinks. With the mind being embodied, the body responds intrinsically from one movement to the next, without any need to stop, judge, or change. Authentic movements, like responding to an itch or stretching the body for a yawn, prompt us to move in response; but the body guides us to understand what we truly need at that moment, perhaps increasing our energy or our rest and recovery. Furthermore, using archetypes/images combined with authentic/natural movement supports the child's physical, emotional, mental, and social well-being. By diving deeper into the unconscious on a physical level, there is potential for transformation (Stromsted, 2009).

Dance/movement therapy provides a space for an active expression of emotional needs and underlying patterns (Stromsted, 2009). Rather than be identified as a formulaic measure that depicts all movements as having one meaning, movement is instead identified as the consistent pattern presented by the individual (child) at particular points (with certain people, within specific environments, during relevant emotional/psychological or medical states of development). Therefore, the provider (therapist) or a parent can bring a connection to these movements and have a direct lens into the embodied experience of the individual (child). This also allows for authentic connection and treatment based on what is happening at that moment instead of what is expected or as a product-based outcome. As related to the "Surviving the Volcano" (Chapter 1, Vignette 3), research studies have examined the interplay of memory, problem-solving, and imagination in people with depression. These studies revealed that episodic memory and imagination both use the same neural structures, which may mean that imagination and memory lead to problem-solving and a broad range of cognitive activities (McFarland, Primosch, Maxson, & Stewart, 2017).

Qualities of Movement

The child's movement can be broken down into effort qualities (such as the way in which a child moves within their body, and with interactions between others), including the speed of movement (quick or slow pace) or the weightedness of the body (such as heaviness or lightness within their hand gestures or shoulder posture), directional patterns (described as how a child moves from one point to another or takes up the environmental space to include multiple directions at one time), and awareness (mindfulness). Movement analysis is a method and language for describing, visualizing, interpreting, and documenting all varieties of human motion; movement studies identify consistent patterns and qualities of motion across humankind. In my clinical practice the lens of reading the child's movements and interpreting through these qualities, patterns and awarenesses has informed my understanding and connection to the child's emotional state and needs. Furthermore, allowing the child and parents to learn the lens of

DMT provides a new skill set for them to build a relationship that fosters acceptance for the physicality of emotional regulation.

Timing can be seen as a critical instrument in which all relationships are met with congruency, fluidity, synchronicity, disruption, hostility, intensity, and even chaos. Timing also pertains to how quickly or slowly a child moves, in singular and gross movements, independently or within a relationship. In a child's movement patterns, the body weaves through an environment with intentionality, toward a specific stimulus or away from it; there is also focus on the direct relationship with the person/place/object so as to take in more area and multiple objects/individuals at once.

As for space, a common example of what characterizes this effort quality is the difference between a child popping one bubble versus watching all the bubbles float in the air. And the effort quality of weight, or use of the body against gravity, presents another expression of movement indicated by emotional/psychological states and health: A child lacking purpose and resilience may be seen as without weight as if the body is drifting; a child with presence and connection can be seen as balanced and unencumbered; a child with too much heaviness in posture and body movement may appear held down and depleted; conversely, a child light on their feet and disconnected may seem hard to grasp or non-compliant and aloof (Tsachor & Shafir, 2017).

The D.A.N.C.E.

Using this method, we assess motion against a background of planes of movement: Horizontal, vertical, and sagittal. As depicted in the Chapter 1 vignettes and provided in the intervention strategies, the planes of movement can support the therapeutic needs of children in their development and relationships (Chaiklin & Wengrower, 2015).

The interventions of using the planes of movement facilitate the embodiment of repairing and building a foundation for interaction. Again, the child is provided with a space to move gradually through the developmental stages of growth and connection. This exploration of movement offers expanded opportunities for increasing timing with the speed of motions; development of weight with qualities of heaviness, strength, and lightness; and directionality for moving within the body, in connection to another, and through the environmental space.

With attachment as our main organizing principle, movement becomes the transitional object that connects the child to the provider or parent. Movement may be expressed through the entire body, also with props and objects that bring a more meaningful connection to emotional expression and therapeutic goals. These movement activities can be repeated, or a child may stay in one pattern of movement for a while before comfortably shifting to the next – and ultimately through – each range of motion. The dance/movement therapy lens will be addressed in further detail throughout this book and in the final chapter's use of dance/movement therapy in application.

For clinical practice, I invite everyone to use the dance/movement therapy lens to understand the full dance of connectedness – integration stems from differentiated parts that are linked together (Siegel, 2018). We can use DANCE (see Figure 3.10) as an acronym to mean Differentiation, Attachment, Narration, Consciousness, and Empathic Engagement, a method that applies to all interactions. DANCE encourages integration, therapeutic alliance, and practical application in each clinical context, and we use effort qualities, dimensional planes, authentic movement, imaginary exploration, and more dance/movement therapy methods within the DANCE of each session.

To start the dance/movement therapy interaction, I always focus on differentiation (D) so each child's movement has a separate function and purpose. When I observe the child's individualized movements, I consider the patterns, celebrate intentions, and come to understand the distinctions and unique nature of the child. I then attach (A) these movements together to form phrases, sequences, and interactions, enabling my ability to see the child moving through the environment within these interactions. Narration (N) provides the verbal component needed to bring the child's movements into consciousness (C), in which the child and observing parents

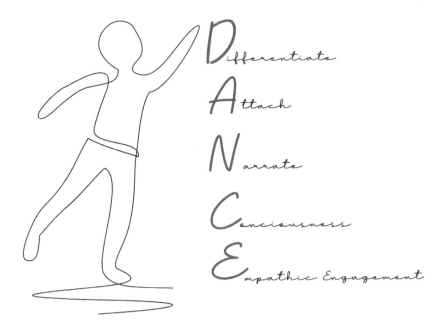

Figure 3.10 DANCE Acronym

learn. Simultaneously, he/she/they experience empathic engagement (E) when a sense of being truly seen and accepted develops, allowing for clinical care and meaningful connection.

DANCE is an effective lens through which we can slow down and wholly grasp the connections formed by the therapeutic alliance while acting as a framework inherent to each interaction. DANCE is always a part of communication style, family dynamics, therapeutic relationships, and the healing process. These movement observation skills can immediately bring attunement into the therapeutic relationship and family dynamics. This further supports myriad connections to the vastness of our displayed movements and life patterns.

Clinical Integration of DMT for the Whole Child

Now, when considering the etiology of ASD and neurodivergence, (as indicated earlier), and the movement profiles of children with anxiety and pain (from Chapter 2), you are better informed to support the whole child. You can use the dance/movement therapy lens to understand each moving moment vignette presented throughout this book and apply these practices in your interactions with children. Keep in mind to:

- Observe when the body appears calm and alert (integration/regulation).
- Recognize the lack of core stability (whether the child sits in a "W" position when on the ground and other indicators of weakened postural control, including the mouth and tongue in breathing).
- Notice when you see restrictions such as tightened muscles, a flat facial affect, direct movements from point A to B, and preferences for linear play with familiar patterns and outcomes (rigidity).
- Notice when you see asymmetry and reactive movements such as flailing arms, limp head posture, indirect motions, and drifting/floating motions without intention (chaos).
- Acknowledge whether the individual prefers moving side to side in rocking or forward and back (dimensional planes).

These observations will enable you to support the child amid potential chaos, rigidity, and disconnection to a place of integration and connection. A child may present with movement preferences, so it's important to note when the movement pattern does not match the interactions, expectations of the environment, or needs of the individual. Provide support for effective movement expression, such as when a child can enact free, chaotic movements outside in an open space versus moving in this manner within a classroom setting. Supporting a child to be intentional and aware of his/her/their movements, the etiquette of the set environment, and the child's individual needs further invite health and healing. After you become familiar with assessing preferred movement styles, you may join the child and try their way of moving. Practice with your body – see what you feel and notice.

With an understanding of varying degrees of etiology, how to guide discussion for best practices for your individual child, and some initial steps for observation and connection, you have an expanded lens through which to value the purpose symptoms serve and better experience the capabilities and resilience of each individual.

Thankfully, all this focus on the body allows for an integrative experience within the child that fosters optimal health.

> Dance/movement therapy may be conceptualized as an embodied and enactive form of psychotherapy. The embodied enactive approach looks at individuals as *living* systems characterized by plasticity and permeability (moment-to-moment adaptations within the self and toward the environment), autonomy, sense-making, emergence, experience, and striving for balance. Enaction and embodiment emphasize the roles that body motion and sensorimotor experience play in the formation of concepts and abstract thinking.
>
> (Koch & Fischman, 2011, p. 1)

References

Americandancemovement.org/health-initiative

Arky, B. (2023). *Twice-exceptional kids: Both gifted and challenged.* Childmind.org/artice/twice-exceptional-kids-both-gifted-and-challenged

Birkland, M. F. (2007). *The effect of the DIR/Floortime model on communication in children with autism.* Washington State University.

Chaiklin, S., & Wengrower, H. (2015). *The art and science of dance/movement therapy: Life is dance.* Routledge.

Cordero, J., Greenspan, S. I., Bauman, M. L., Brazelton, T. B., Dawson, G., Dunbar, B., Mundy, P. C., Perou, R., Scott, K. G., Shanker, S. G., & Others. (2006). *CDC/ICDL collaboration report on a framework for early identification and preventive intervention of emotional and developmental challenges.* The Centers for Disease Control.

Delahooke, M. (2019). *Beyond behaviors: Using brain science and compassion to understand and solve children's behavioral challenges.* PESI Publishing & Media.

Gagliano, A., Carta, A., Tanca, M. G., & Sotgiu, S. (2023). Pediatric acute-onset neuropsychiatric syndrome: Current perspectives. *Neuropsychiatric Disease and Treatment, 19,* 1221–1250. https://doi.org/10.2147/NDT.S362202

Greenspan, S. I., & Wieder, S. (2007). The developmental individual-difference, relationship-based (DIR/Floortime) model approach to autism spectrum disorders. In E. Hollander & E. Anagnostou (Eds.), *Clinical manual for the treatment of autism* (pp. 179–209). American Psychiatric Publishing, Inc.

Heyes, C. (2010). Where do mirror neurons come from? *Neuroscience & Biobehavioral Reviews, 34*(4), 575–583.

Kattenstroth, J.-C., Kalisch, T., Holt, S., Tegenthoff, M., & Dinse, H. R. (2013). Six months of dance intervention enhances postural, sensorimotor, and cognitive performance in elderly without affecting cardio-respiratory functions. *Frontiers in Aging Neuroscience*, 5, 5.

Koch, S. C., & Fischman, D. (2011). Embodied enactive dance/movement therapy. *American Journal of Dance Therapy*, 33(1), 57–72.

Maté, G. (2011). *When the body says no: The cost of hidden stress.* Knopf Canada.

Mavilidi, M. F., Pesce, C., Benzing, V., Schmidt, M., Paas, F., Okely, A. D., & Vazou, S. (2022). Meta-analysis of movement-based interventions to aid academic and behavioral outcomes: A taxonomy of relevance and integration. *Educational Research Review*, 37, 100478.

McFarland, C. P., Primosch, M., Maxson, C. M., & Stewart, B. T. (2017). Enhancing memory and imagination improves problem solving among individuals with depression. *Memory & Cognition*, 45(6), 932–939.

Najafabadi, M. G., Sheikh, M., Hemayattalab, R., Memari, A. H., Aderyani, M. R., & Hafizi, S. (2018). The effect of spark on social and motor skills of children with autism. *Pediatrics and Neonatology*, 59(5), 481–487.

Rafiei Milajerdi, H., Sheikh, M., Najafabadi, M. G., Saghaei, B., Naghdi, N., & Dewey, D. (2021). The effects of physical activity and exergaming on motor skills and executive functions in children with autism spectrum disorder. *Games for Health Journal*, 10(1), 33–42.

Siegel, D. (2018). *Aware: The science and practice of presence: The groundbreaking meditation practice.* Penguin.

Silverman, M., Frankovich, J., Nguyen, E., Leibold, C., Yoon, J., Mark Freeman, G., Jr, Karpel, H., & Thienemann, M. (2019). Psychotic symptoms in youth with Pediatric Acute-Onset Neuropsychiatric Syndrome (PANS) may reflect syndrome severity and heterogeneity. *Journal of Psychiatric Research*, 110, 93–102. https://doi.org/10.1016/j.jpsychires.2018.11.013

Stromsted, T. (2009). Authentic movement: A dance with the divine. *Body, Movement and Dance in Psychotherapy*, 4(3), 201–213. https://doi.org/10.1080/17432970902913942

Tsachor, R. P., & Shafir, T. (2017). A somatic movement approach to fostering emotional resiliency through Laban movement analysis. *Frontiers in Human Neuroscience*, 11, 410.

Voss, P., Thomas, M. E., Cisneros-Franco, J. M., & de Villers-Sidani, E. (2019). Dynamic brains and the changing rules of neuroplasticity: Implications for learning and recovery. *Frontiers in Psychology*, 8, 1657. Retrieved November 24, 2019. www.ncbi.nlm.nih.gov/pmc/articles/PMC5649212/

Wieder, S., & Greenspan, S. I. (2003). Climbing the symbolic ladder in the DIR model through floor time/interactive play. *Autism: The International Journal of Research and Practice*, 7(4), 425–435.

Chapter 4

Everyday Life With Kids – Siblings, Identities, and Behaviors

Vignette 1: Family Moves

"I miss my family."

– Sophia, age 14

Sophia's hospital room was filled with photos and cards from her family members. She led me around her space and introduced me to each person who "cared for her." She smiled when I asked her how each person typically moved, and she immediately made a gesture, a pose, and a phrase that captured each person.

Sophia had five siblings, parents, three grandparents, and four cousins. She knew what each person meant to her. She used wide stances to characterize some of them and smaller, more subtle movements for others (to indicate her grandmother, she pressed her palms together, wiggled her fingers, and bent over in prayer). She also identified which family members seemed the most similar and which seemed more different (for her father and brother, she made a stomping motion, as if they were marching in place, versus her mother and youngest sibling swaying side to side).

Sophia began to move in a sequenced pattern like a dance routine as if her family were right there in the room with her. Each person was represented by motion within the movement pattern she had designated for them ("My mom sways, my dad stomps, my grandmother prays" etc.).

Tears welled up in her eyes as she slowed the routine down and performed it in front of me again. Each family member had become a part of her own embodied experience. She then invited me to watch her way of moving: She stretched out farther than any family member had moved, grabbing toward her "perceived family members," and pulling her arms toward her body in a strong embrace – as if she had all her family in the room hugging her. Lastly, she invited me to show her a movement to represent myself. I gently floated my arms out toward her, we connected our hands to one another and smiled. She then told me I was among those who cared for her.

DOI: 10.4324/9781003363491-5

> ### *Vignette 1 Intervention:* Family Moves
>
> **Activity Prompt:** Explore with the child the following prompt: Getting to know the family. Create a movement for each person in your family. What would they look like if they moved? (How would they move their hands? Would they move quickly or slowly)?

Provider Note: *Ensure this is a safe movement exploration for each participant. Everyone agrees to participate individually, and the child shares one-on-one with the provider. The movements can be fully active or stationary postures/poses. The activity can take the form of charades in enacting how the family member moves. Discuss patterns, preferences, and desires. Take an opportunity to invite gratitude into the discussion. Have parents acknowledge and reflect on the child's strengths and growth points.*

Vignette 2: Kaleidoscope Play

"That boy is so rude when he tells me what to do. I told him to stop it."
— Brian, age 7

When a parent or child communicates a strong belief, judgment, or a label for describing another person, I think about a kaleidoscope. When we look at ourselves and each other like a simple cylinder of colors tilted to one side or the other, it reveals an entirely different picture and perspective. As adults, we tend to label specific actions and movements with judgmental words like "rude," "aggressive," "lazy," "bossy," and "shy." We may see the situation from one angle, but a child could have a completely different perspective and might just be moving. I acknowledge behaviors as movements rather than definitive intentions or states of being.

In therapy, when Brian told me about his classmate's rudeness, I supported him to first look at his own body posture, facial expression, and tension in his muscle movements. We explored what his body state communicated through his "kaleidoscope." Then we observed his classmate's body movements and postures. Brian laughed as he shook his stiff shoulders and shared that he and the classmate had the same tight muscle posture. He realized that neither of them was rude but was just displaying a tense posture that could easily be changed or shaken off.

This new perspective on the movement made Brian feel more inclusive of his classmate's needs, ultimately opening his awareness to accept his friend as more like him than different. The new, or changed, image in the kaleidoscope showed two boys trying to navigate a new friendship – two boys being assertive and engaging, not "rude."

Vignette 2 Intervention: Kaleidoscope Play

Activity Prompt: Explore with the child the following prompt: Take a posture and move it. Try your friends or classmates' movements/postures and notice similarities and differences. Write down a label and how it looks in movement. Explore verbally how the "behavior" is just a body movement, try to omit your assumptions or judgments.

Provider Note: *Remember, perspective-taking is about noticing that behaviors are just movement choices and adaptive responses. Using movement with a partner promotes more understanding and connection. Try and encourage a commonality or uniqueness to everyone's movements.*

Vignette 3: The Movement Experiment

> *"This child doesn't say much or cause any distractions."*
> — Teacher of Billy, age 13

The alarm bells go off when we see or hear a child acting out – raising his voice, pushing his body, or disrupting his class. But what about the quiet kids that tend to be overlooked?

When Billy woke up in the morning, he took a while to get energized. In therapy, he said he felt lonely and disconnected, like "his body was asleep."

When I observed Billy at school, I noticed that he was easily missed. He didn't call much attention to himself. He was able to go with the flow of the day, yet he had limited interactions with the other children and teachers at school.

I noticed that when he walked down the street, the people he passed didn't look at him. They didn't say hello or make eye contact. I counted ten different people, including children and adults, who passed by him without acknowledgement. I realized the detrimental impact that these social situations had on Billy's mental health and how imperative it was to support his body movements to promote connection and well-being.

Billy and I decided that, while it wouldn't be easy, he was going to create a social experiment. Using the body postures, gestures, and facial affect we had practiced, he would try to elicit a simple wave or nod from the people who passed him.

On Monday, he attempted this movement experiment. Within the first ten minutes of being dropped off at school, he said that one out of the five adults he nodded at responded with a smile. The other four didn't even see him. He initially reported feeling discouraged, mixed with a feeling of familiarity with this lack of attention. But he started to realize that, despite his lack of control over others, he actually had control over himself, especially his body movements.

Within a week, he had increased the number of positive responses by moving faster, lifting his head higher, and adding a smile. He was able to raise people's awareness of him and, in turn, he communicated that he felt more awake and alive.

This simple movement challenge provided Billy with insight into his interactions and the effects his body choices had on his relationships. When he connected socially with other people, he expressed feeling happier and more a part of his school.

Vignette 3 Intervention: The Movement Experiment

Activity Prompt: Explore with the child the following movement prompt and questions: Explore using your body movements, gestures, and facial expressions when greeting someone. Do you notice how they respond and how you feel? Take the movement experiment and see how many people acknowledge you.

Provider Note: *Ensure safety by starting the movement exploration with one another and then with close family or friends. Explore verbally various possibilities of reactions when greeting other people. Explore context-specific differences and socially accepted practices (i.e., welcoming in a library versus at a park). Emphasize the importance of movement greetings and how to initiate transitions by encouraging care providers to recognize and respond to a child's movements.*

Vignette 4: Movement Conquers Bad Dreams

"I have bad dreams and bad thoughts."

– Max, age 7

Max sat calmly in his hospital bed under his covers. His dad sat next to him silently reading a book. Neither one was talking or interacting with the other. I asked Max what was up. "I can't sleep because I have bad thoughts and dreams," he said. Meanwhile, his father continued to read. I asked Max if he could remember his thoughts from a dream and whether we could explore them together.

We did. We moved, made faces, and re-created his dream. His dad heard our laughter and looked up to see what we were doing. I invited him to join us and follow Max's movements, which he did. The two of them flashed through wild and twisted poses and scrunched up their faces as if they were creeping up on each other (just like Max had seen in his dream and had felt in his body). I asked them to move on from these images to something opposite, small, soft, straight, calm, and then to something larger and stronger.

Together, they decided to move at the same time with slow but strong postures. Their eyes met and they hugged. Max said he didn't feel scared anymore because his dad was with him now and he could share his experience with him.

Movement exploration between parents and children can unlock confusion and support a child's need for problem-solving tools and resolution. Therapeutic support with movement can be powerful for children who are otherwise unable to communicate uncomfortable topics and fears.

Vignette 4 Intervention: Movement Conquers Bad Dreams

Activity Prompt: Explore with the child the following prompt: Combat nighttime dreams. Write out your dreams (or have a parent write for you) and then express them in movement. Explore together the feelings and qualities of the dream scenario when expressed through the movement experiential.

Provider Note: *Support each idea experienced in the dream by role-playing and moving. Ask if the timing, weight, and use of space feel similar or different from the dream. Support the child to fill in missing parts by adding movement and building the movement story (phrase/routine). Incorporate writing, drawing, or talking.*

Vignette 5: Transform a Child in Your Life

"Our child needs support. She won't look or communicate with people."
— Mother of Olivia, age 4

Olivia was a four-year-old child diagnosed on the autism spectrum. She used repetitive hitting behaviors, appeared to have little awareness of others, and could not access words or make eye contact.

To engage with Olivia, I imagined building a castle for a princess. I imagined building the castle's structure: First, the frame must be established horizontally, just as our relationship would need to have a foundation and sense of comfort. Next, the walls had to be set up vertically to give the castle a sturdy stature – again, like our individual stance and presence in our environment. Finally, the drawbridge, which needed to open and close sagittally to welcome only the kindest suitors; specifically, our connection would strengthen and enable her to communicate with me in a secure, trusting relationship.

The session structure followed this order too: We started with horizontal movement and sat in two separate areas of the room. Olivia placed any items she'd found (shoes, toys, scarves) around her, like the foundation's walls. She seemed to be protecting herself in a new territory. I paralleled this on my side, mirroring and reflecting her actions. In time, she initiated vertical and sagittal movement. She stood up and peeked over her walls. We explored each other's space and moved with the same rhythm and timing. She reached out and pressed our hands together, connecting with me and allowing me to join her across her castle walls. We joined our spaces together and danced. We made eye contact! We laughed! She went from hitting walls and her body to using the same rhythm to build, share, and connect without hitting.

The emphasis on timing (using the pattern of her preferred hitting to create a movement to safely connect), the analogy of the castle, and the dance/movement therapy planes of movement (horizontal, vertical, sagittal) enabled me to engage with Olivia. Ultimately, she made sounds, and we created new rituals in which she could anticipate my actions. This eventually led to further learning and problem-solving for her.

Often, with a child identified on the autism spectrum, experts talk about finding a gleam in the child's eyes the moment when a connection is made. By utilizing body knowledge to move within these specific movement planes and joining this child as if moving up a developmental ladder, I could then make progress and find that gleam shining through.

Vignette 5 Intervention: **Transform a Child in Your Life**

Activity Prompt: Model the following movement patterns and explore the prompt within the clinical sessions: Start in the horizontal plane and move side to side like you're swaying. Then stand up and walk around the room vertically. Then create a connection by moving sagittally with high-fives and holding hands.

Provider Note: *The movement planes invite you to teach and model appropriate and healthy relations. You can link these planes of movement by recalling stories of being held, first steps, and new relationships. Notice how many relational dynamics follow these exact movement dimensions.*

Vignette 6: Can Behaviors Be Ignored?

"Our son is being sent out to the office repeatedly for not joining the class for group tasks and becoming disruptive. Is this typical?"
– Mother of Mathew, age 4

Therapeutic support allows families to explore age-appropriate behaviors, atypical patterns, and, more importantly, the underlying individual differences and needs of their children.

While observing four-year-old Mathew, I became aware of his seemingly melted posture and slow pace during transitions. He appeared overwhelmed and moved away from the group when an unpredicted sound was created by his teacher. When the teacher requested transitioning into group time, she used a different sound such as ringing a chime, singing a song, or clapping her hands. While Mathew cooperated in individual work, his body immediately found ways to create separation and predictability during what he experienced as unpredictable. He developed ritualistic behaviors like looking directly down at his pencil and constantly rubbing his hands on his sides during heightened group dynamics.

Supporting Mathew's sensory needs and regulation required his teacher to set up more consistent transition sounds and create a space where he could, with permission, return as needed so he wouldn't be sent to the office. In sessions, plans were made to practice modulation of sounds and emotional expression amid these uncomfortable feelings. He used movement playfully to explore tones of voice, transitions, and anticipation.

Rather than see Mathew's responses as "bad," the school and family learned how to identify the etiology of his behavior, create opportunities for change, and ultimately expand Mathew's ability to predict and read cues.

Vignette 6 Intervention: **Can Behaviors Be Ignored?**

Activity Prompt: The following prompt can support the clinical sessions: Behaviors can be expressed because of discomfort in your body and with the sensory experiences around you. Simply changing speed or even the use of sounds/volume can support your daily interactions. For instance, do you ever feel like your family is speaking too loud in the morning, or you feel too rushed to get out the door to the car? In this activity, you can explore changing sounds and timing. Think about transitions in your life, for instance leaving the house – can you move quicker out the door, and use a quieter voice when asking your parent for breakfast? Can you notice how the responses and interactions change over the week when you move this way? Ask your parents to try these concepts on at home; can they sing a request to you instead of yelling/demanding? Can they slowly walk to the door instead of rushing you out?

Provider Note: *Remember to keep this straightforward. Notice what is typical, making simple timing shifts (i.e., speed of walking, the cadence of the voice). Discuss, throughout the week, what were the most effective and efficient ways to transition. Write these down to explore patterns over time and best practices for that particular family.*

Vignette 7: Positioning the Sibling Relationship

"What about me? Can I do that too?"

– Bethany, age 5

When you have siblings, you may have competition. Your children will be navigating the many aspects that create their individual differences: academics, athleticism, personality, and even appearance. The slightest facial expression or verbal exchange comparing one sibling to another can lead your child(ren) toward a sense of inequity, the sibling rivalry that comes from asking, "Am I good enough?"

Bethany created a visual picture using toys in the therapy office to indicate her home/school life. She moved each item intentionally and shared how she felt about her brother. She identified her feelings as "jealousy, loss, and even fear."

We connected to this visual display by narrating what we saw in front of us. We discussed how we visually read the scene versus how we felt about it. Bethany noted that her story had her brother in opposition to her toy character. The toy representing her brother was placed up high while her character was low. He had more space while she was bombarded with stuff. At this point, she felt he was "actually" better than her, which gave Bethany a feeling of inadequacy.

We continued to explore the siblings opposite roles. Now, Bethany was able to enjoy her differences, and at other times she saw that she and her brother had a lot in common. For instance, she quickly moved the characters that represented her brother and her; she verbally communicated that both are fast when they play chase together.

The therapeutic environment supported Bethany and her family to become observers rather than just opinionators. They learned to visually identify what was happening instead of labeling situations as either good or bad, better or worse, his or hers. The ability to look at the situation through the lens of movement and positioning allowed Bethany to feel a sense of autonomy and a positive connection to her brother.

Vignette 7 Intervention: Positioning the Sibling Relationship

Activity Prompt: Use the following prompt to explore this theme and bring embodied practices to the clinical session: Choose a toy/object that represents a sibling and one that represents you. Place the object on the floor/table to describe the dynamic between your sibling(s) and you. For example, notice where the toy dog (brother) is placed compared to the toy rabbit (you). Notice if the items are similar or different; if the items are positioned above, below, near, or far. Communicate how you might adjust this picture toward equality and connection.

Provider Note: *The toy/object in this activity symbolizes the child and their sibling(s). The location/positioning of the object invites a safe way to depict the sibling dynamic. Notice movement initiation and timing; does the child move the objects intentionally? Notice if the child pauses or moves quickly through the activity. Discuss and document the exchange for future treatment processing. Relay feedback regarding the symbolic representation and the real-life dynamics.*

Vignette 8: The Three Ps for a Peaceful Holiday

"Why do my children get so out of hand during the holidays . . . jumping, breaking things, screaming, and not listening?"
— Stephanie, mother of three children, ages 2, 5, and 9

Therapeutic support for children means support for their parents and/or care providers too. When Stephanie told me about her family dynamics around the holidays, while her children cheered and jumped around my office, I knew we had to work on the "Three Ps."

Our first session gave the family an opportunity to write, draw, and talk about their favorite holiday memories. Afterward, we sat together and read these memories out loud. We mirrored one another's body postures, facial expressions, and movements. Stephanie jumped like a child, copying her son's favorite way to wake up on a non-school day. By embodying these experiences, Stephanie and her family stopped their judgements and became receptive to the meaningful way the moments physically felt to one another.

We then explored the first P: prune. Pruning means experiencing what is requested and what needs to be gently brushed to the side and changed. For example, Stephanie requested that her family make decisions about the food menu earlier in the week rather than waiting for the last minute; and her son requested they do only one activity outing per day rather than packing in a ton of transitions and events.

The second P stands for preference, meaning understanding the sensory experiences associated with the holidays. What sounds, sights, textures, and smells are preferred? What is not? Again, the family talked, focusing on exploring and moving through feelings. They became aware of their individual sensory needs. We even drew a map to describe which family members were similar and how to use their preferences to create a more peaceful environment at home.

Lastly, the third P stands for practice. Stephanie's family spent several weeks communicating what they wanted to see develop, for example saying, "I admire your sitting so patiently at the table," and "Your voice is loud and playful outside the house."

By exploring these three Ps, each family member got a chance to communicate their needs and ultimately set an expectation for the big holiday moments to come. When changes are coming – whether they're seasons, schedules, expectations, opportunities, or new connections – it's important to explore these areas and make time for the best experiences to take shape. With awareness comes peace!

Vignette 8 Intervention: The Three Ps for a Peaceful Holiday

Activity Prompt: Follow this task to support family holiday dynamics and patterns: Write out the Three Ps – prune, preference, practice – with your parents (and/or in clinical session) before the holiday or upcoming family event. Remember, pruning allows you to think through the areas of the holidays that you don't feel serve you or experiences/interactions/ expectations that do not feel good to you. Your preferences allow you to think even more accurately about the sensory experiences that bring you comfort and joy and those that may feel overwhelming or even upsetting – what sounds do you want to listen to, what odors repel you, or are there any sights that overload your nervouse system? Lastly, practice communicating with your parents and try out new preferences and interactions now that you've locked in what works for you!

Provider Note: *Refer to the vignette to explore the prune, preference, and practice steps for the family before the family event/holiday. Encourage discussion and movement exploration, such as mindfulness breathing and authentic movement, to invite the child/family to embody these situations and truly identify their patterns and needs.*

Vignette 9: Understanding a Child's Needs

> *"I just want to make him happy, but now he doesn't use words. He only whines to get things."*
>
> – Mother of Raj, age 4

Raj constantly whined and cried the moment someone walked into his room. He presented with a delay in expressive language, and disparity between his intellectual, receptive processing, and emotional functioning. He often sat on the ground and grunted while gesturing toward what he wanted. If he had to wait, he became upset and fell backward, arching his back and head. His mother was at a loss. She just wanted to make him happy, and therefore immediately accommodated his requests without waiting for him to use clear words, movements, or modeling for him to use words.

I encouraged his mother to take five minutes to observe and follow Raj's movements. I wanted her to be able to slow down and start to anticipate his needs before he complained. When she mirrored her son's movements (joining him on the floor, rolling a toy car back and forth like he was doing), he stopped crying. I supported Raj's mother in observing the timing, patterns, and weight of his actions. By starting with nonverbal communication, we were able to match his needs and increase his ability to express himself verbally.

I acknowledged that Raj's mother was joining her son in parallel play. This developmentally appropriate exchange created an opportunity for connection. In return, Raj increased his movements. When he looked up, he started to cry for us to open a small bag of toys; instead of doing it for him, though, I supported his mother by saying – with facial affect, voice tone, and gesture – "OPPPPPENNNNN!" We opened our hands and signed "open" to him, which sustained his tolerance for waiting and supported his ability to independently achieve his needs. Pairing words with movement increased his understanding and trust in his mother's response. Raj looked at both of us, laughed, and also opened his hands. He repeated the word back to us for the first time.

When a child's movements are shared, seen, and supported, he/she/they may start to communicate verbally. In Raj's case, we joined the child's language of nonverbal movement to enable him to join our language of words.

Vignette 9 Intervention: Understanding a Child's Needs

Activity Prompt: Explore the following prompt and model the examples provided during the clinical session: Provide an opportunity to change words into actions. Move through a task or challenge with a parent or the provider. They will be offering a response to your challenge by using playful obstruction (i.e., rather than solving for you, the provider or parent will join you in your struggle and ultimately have you solve the task).

Provider Note: *This activity explores a child's moment of challenge or need for help. You are modeling how to encourage independence and joining versus helping, enabling, or solving for them. Bringing your facial expression, posturing, and even words that say what you see happening will create further autonomy and resolution. For example: Imagine the jar is tough to open. Pass the jar back and forth until the child opens it independently. Then exchange a word, facial expression, or gesture.*

Vignette 10: Opening Space for New Beginnings

"I don't want to go back to school."

– Roland, age 7

Most of you have heard this quote from your children, or even have your own similar memory of not wanting to return to school, transition from the weekend, or attend a class online or in person. What is it about *not* wanting to go? Is it really about the event or place, or is it something else?

By utilizing strategies to support movement and the body, Roland and I were able to explore exactly what he meant. Roland's body posture, timing of movements, and intentions during our summer sessions were indulgent. He leisurely walked into the room, slowly made his decisions, and felt no pressure as we connected.

I met him in his moment-to-moment state. During this session, as he paced and rushed to fit in everything he had in mind, he questioned whether he was okay to say what he was saying. I acknowledged the change in his timing and body posture. He was able to identify this as a feeling of "frustration" and "pressure." He said, "I'm losing time. Summer is over."

Together, we decided to explore time through our movements. We moved quickly and then slowly, all while discussing memories of Roland's summers and his school years. When he was engaged at a fast pace, he exhibited tension in his muscles, tightness in his facial affect, and rigidity in his movements. But he then realized that moving quickly actually felt freeing and energizing. Together, we acknowledged that he ultimately had a choice of how to experience the movement of his body.

We concluded our session by discussing with Roland's parents his request for more time and support during this transition back to school. His parents

---

Vignette 10 Intervention: Opening Space for New Beginnings

Activity Prompt: The provider will introduce the following embodied practices by engaging in the movement activity provided: Begin by standing on one side of the room. Challenge one another to see how to get to the other side. First, see if you and the provider can go in slow motion. Pay attention to every part of the body moving slowly (i.e., place the tips of the toes down onto the ground as you roll your foot, making contact with the ground before lifting again). Each step is slower than the next. What are the feelings, images, or memories evoked by the slow pace? Once you get to the other side, discuss. Next, turn around, and change the speed to quickness to see how fast you can make it to the other side. Write or discuss when these qualities of time and space are used in daily life.

Provider Note: *Depending on the child's profile you can choose the order in which you go fast or slow. Sometimes, you may start with the child's preference of moving quickly and then revert to slowness or vice versa. Pay attention to these patterns as they may indicate the child's patterns in society or their home. Exploring themes and feelings connected to this activity invites further discussion and therapeutic exploration.*

supported his needs and communicated their own needs for transferring the ease of summer into their daily lives during the academic year.

By examining his body and movement, Roland could connect the emotional experience of transitioning to school to his ability to embody change and comfort. Additionally, the parents and child could communicate about their needs and make plans for a successful new beginning.

Vignette 11: Elevate Your Child

"How do I get my children to stop fighting? Every time they start to play, they become so competitive and appear to want so much attention."
– Father of two children, ages 6 and 4

Six-year-old Patty got into fights with her younger brother daily over her toys. Her parents communicated how these interactions became so distressing that the two kids screamed, pulled hair, and even hit each other. The parents felt that they needed to take the toys away from the house. This was met with more heartbreak and upset.

In session, I supported the family and Patty to understand her needs and how she could obtain physical space for her toys while collaborating with her brother. First, we addressed questions regarding the dynamic between Patty and her brother, the space available for her to play, and her interests in playing. We explored the various rooms she could play in with her toys, and why she felt the common space was most desirable. We wondered why she often "bragged" to her brother and competed with him. She expressed her fears about messing up, losing toy pieces, or her brother taking over and receiving more attention than her. Ultimately, Patty wanted praise for her creative ideas, and she wanted her brother and parents to see her for who she was: "Creative, smart, and fun," she said. Her worries and concerns led to big reactions and meltdowns. Additionally, we looked at her tone of voice, posture, and mannerisms. The therapeutic setting assessed days of upsets and simplified them for a solution that, with practice, worked for everyone.

Patty considered what her brother could do to join her in play instead of telling him, "No!" We created a plan for organizing the set-up of the activity and the space in which it occurred. We even broke the tasks down to make them more manageable and rewarding. Previously, playtime felt too unstructured and overwhelming.

Patty recognized that she could play cooperatively with her brother and her toys. Knowing she could talk things out with her brother enabled her to calm down. She no longer feared the threat of having her toys taken away or that her brother would have more attention from her parents. This meant not only more playtime but also a better relationship with her brother. Her parents recognized her efforts and praised Patty for her collaboration and play ideas. Her family home felt less combative and upsetting – and her parents promised her toys could stay!

Vignette 11 Intervention: Elevate Your Child

Activity Prompt: Explore the following prompt: Creating space. Identify how many areas to use for collaborative play versus independent play. Can you choose toys to share and play with your siblings or friends? Explore how your body posture can be receptive/dismissive for connecting with a sibling or peer. Model posturing for receptive versus dismissive communication. Can you notice which posture is more inviting?

Provider Note: *When you explore these concepts with the child, use "movement" words, such as open or closed instead of receptive/dismissive, to evoke an embodied understanding. When you practice these postures, omit judgment, and notice your interpretations of these movements. Invite exploration and discussion.*

Vignette 12: Transform Your Parenting Experience

"His favorite thing to do was jump, but he can't jump anymore."
– Father of Josh, age 3

I stood beside a child lying in bed in his hospital room. His parents stood across from me. Josh was just three years old and unable to move on his own. He attentively listened to his parents' words, appearing interested in an opportunity to explore movement, while unsure how that would be possible.

After Josh's parents talked about his joys, I offered a way for us to move together, hoping to transform the seemingly impossible into something doable. To start, I had the parents gently tap on their son's body, beginning with his feet. They did this with a rhythm like a heartbeat as if they were saying "hello" to each part of Josh's body, perhaps to wake him and connect to him. The child lay still with a smile on his face and then verbally responded: Glancing down at his body, he softly said, "Hello," back and watched as his parents acknowledged him in full. Josh's parents, with his permission, then each took a leg and gently lifted it up in the air and down again. Each time we sang "Up" his parents lifted his legs up, always gently. The boy giggled and laughed, saying, "More."

Josh's parents stood with tears in their eyes and continued the song and movements. A connection was created, and a new possibility emerged. The parents said they felt their son's muscles tighten, and he really seemed like he was jumping. They all had fun.

Afterward, we were able to talk about memories and changes. This was such a simple moment of pleasure, worth every second. Within the therapeutic space, the family was offered the choice to bring knowledge to the body and to connect. This is a choice that all children have, even those with physical mobility issues: The ability to move within, between, or with another.

Vignette 12 Intervention: Transform Your Parenting Experience

Activity Prompt: Explore, model, and provide the following movement opportunity within the clinical session: Start with the limbs (arms/legs), and with your permission, have the provider gently tap or provide appropriate input to each part of your body (as if saying hello to each toe, foot, etc.). Next, share a memory related to that part of your body and then create a moving story about that memory.

Provider Note: *The initial tapping is a way to help the child become alert and ready to start verbal communication. The child can complete this activity independently, or you may guide the parent to provide the physical input and movement choices while you guide them through the exercise. The child may be sitting or standing.*

Vignette 13: Helpful Hands

"Stop telling me what to do! I am not your personal assistant."
          – Rachel, mother of three children, ages 5, 8, and 11

This moving moment provides understanding and strategies to support mothers, parents, and care providers with all their hard work. Do your kids help at home?

Rachel wondered how to teach her children to help around the house. She needed them to stop requesting everything from her and instead be able to get their own food, clothes, clean their dishes, etc. While smiling, she would ask her children to complete a task; however, she had tense shoulders and even raised her voice. And yet her children did not respond.

By adopting methods that support using the whole body, the family started to work together. Instead of requesting a task, Rachel would state what she saw with her eyes: "I see you are sitting at the table with your dirty plate. Now we will put our plates in the sink." The entire family stood up, moved to the sink, and then to the family room. Rachel acknowledged that verbally stating the movement patterns and visual aspects of the situations, then actively moving through the process, created ease and acceptance. She started initiating games. "Let's see how fast we can pick up the blue blocks, how slowly we can brush our teeth, how tall we can walk to the door, and how heavy we can push our bodies into bed," she'd say.

The use of these phrases and actions created exploration, playfulness, and learning. Her children saw the tasks as meaningful opportunities to engage and connect with their mom. Instead of connecting only through a demand, they now had other options to be together.

Vignette 13 Intervention: Helpful Hands

Activity Prompt: Within the clinical session, complete the following activity prompt and questions: Write down three parental demands that have been placed on you (i.e., go to bed, pick up your clothes). Identify the manner (what does this action look like in your body?) of how you can complete that demand/task. Now, practice with the provider in different ways you could move through the demand/task. For example, "Go to bed!" How? Run or tiptoe to bed, slow, rush, crawl, or hop.

Provider Note: *The demands are the parental expectations that the parents ask the child to complete daily or weekly. The focus of this activity is to acknowledge the "how" (i.e., the child completes the task/demand physically in their body movements and facial affect) and promote shared control of the expectation. By inviting playful and purposeful movement, the child can master the task and find joy and a meaningful connection to the daily routine.*

Vignette 14: Finding Joy

"Is she always happy? She is so much fun to be with and she is always smiling!"
— Sophia, age 4

Sophia, with her smile, curly ponytail, and energetic nature, was seen as a typical four-year-old girl. She had a lot to say and seemed eager to join most activities, especially if she had her friends with her. Her father brought her to therapy because, even though Sophia acted happy and engaged in public, at home she showed a lot of big feelings – feelings he often had no clue how to handle. He was concerned.

On a weekly basis, I heard stories of Sophia's ups and downs. When her father repeated a demand or tried to teach her something (a seemingly harmless intention), he was unaware that this made Sophia feel like he didn't believe she was smart or capable. His assertiveness appeared overpowering to her smaller, cute stature. Sophia responded best when her father was more curious and collaborative in his exchanges, getting on her level physically, and using a playful facial affect to encourage a connection.

In therapy, Sophia learned how to be aware of the big feelings in her body. She role-played situations in which she would have to problem-solve without becoming angry or reverting to screaming at her dad. Sophia also learned about regulation and how to organize her body to read her father's facial cues and *attend* to his words versus reacting to a perceived threat (her father's quality of assertive movement).

Sophia felt comfortable when she was able to share control and participate in activities that allowed her to move. For instance, she explored using her physical strength (how to stand tall, open a secure toy box, and carry a chair with her dad) and when to initiate lightness (passing a toy, walking

---

Vignette 14 Intervention: Finding Joy

Activity Prompt: Complete the following activity during the clinical sessions or provide the activity for parent/child to try at home: Take a moment to explore facial affect/expressions with the provider or your parents. Can we guess your feelings just by looking at your face? Now expand to the whole body. What posture do you use to show you are playing? How do you move when you are busy? Practice together to find a typical movement pattern for your family and you during different feelings/feeling states. Now have the provider or your parents do this activity and try to guess their feelings in different scenarios.

> **Provider Note:** *You can use a mirror to explore this activity. You can use this activity with one child or their whole family to develop movement preferences and profiles. For example, this could look like the game charades. (How does mom move? How does dad move? How does your kid move?) Each family member takes turns acting out each other. Additionally, this activity can promote awareness for the child to know how he/she/they look to others when displaying feelings or completing a task.*

up to her father, sharing an idea). Through intentional movement, she gained a better understanding of the impact she had on others, especially her dad. Sophia practiced relaxing and playing games, like movement charades, with her dad to better communicate and read social cues. Most importantly, Sophia and her dad learned more about each other, and how to trust each other, which helped them learn how to cope with their differences. Sophia's dad felt joyful that he and his daughter could be friends. Getting to know children allows them to get to know us.

Vignette 15: Honoring Space

> *"I feel a ball of rage inside of me."*
> — Mac, age 17 (identifies as nonbinary; pronouns they/them)

Mac entered the session feeling anxious and overwhelmed. I observed their overall posture and body language: Shoulders concave, head/neck extended forward, and hips/pelvis jutting outward. Mac came to therapy having been diagnosed with autism, ADHD, anxiety, agoraphobia, and trauma. They had revealed experiences of troubling family dynamics and the struggle of sharing their gender identity.

Mac had attended therapy for four months with a focused goal to unpack their relational themes and bring personal acceptance to their gender identity. The therapeutic alliance was quickly felt as Mac expressed feeling safe in my way of sitting, which matched their stance and provided consistent timing, breathing, and space within the room. Mac shared their identity as nonbinary and requested the use of they/them pronouns, preferring to go by Mac instead of their birth name. Getting the opportunity to establish pronouns, a preferred name, and related language was recognized by Mac as a novel and refreshing experience.

During one of our sessions, Mac walked into the therapy room and communicated that they had very high anxiety that day and a list of things to discuss. I asked if, first, we could explore some movement and breathing exercises to help reduce the anxiety before talking. Mac agreed and put down their backpack. We began by rubbing our hands together, creating friction (our energy), closing our eyes, and breathing deeply. Then Mac slowly moved their hands away, felt the energy that they created, and tapped it from their legs all the way up to their head. We began shaking our different body parts and then shook everything together. We stretched to the right and left and swung our arms horizontally from side to side. We stretched out our arms up to the sky and then down to the ground. The movement differentiated our body parts and connected the whole body in alignment and full expansive release.

As we rolled up through our body to an upright posture, I invited Mac to follow what movement felt good to them. They continued to rock side to side with their arms wrapped around their body like a hug. I asked if Mac would be open to me following them and joining in this movement, and they agreed. The movement was slow at first, then quickened. The side-to-side movement appeared soothing and safe. I invited Mac to take up as much preferred space in the room. I secured this moment by moving in the same way as Mac, which was to get as small as we could and then expand our arms and legs and reach around us. We continued to move inward and outward for a few minutes (I could see Mac's body finding alignment and connection through their initial body stance from the start of our session). The movement became a complete expression, moving around the room, increasing space, and utilizing the whole body in relation to themselves and me. Ultimately, we slowed down to stillness, and Mac placed their hands on their heart and stomach and closed their eyes. The movement experience concluded with Mac giving their body a self-hug and sitting down comfortably to talk. Mac reflected on how their anxious feelings had dissipated as we moved and then were released with their final hug and breath.

Mac acknowledged that they felt initial discomfort when transitioning from starting small to gradually taking up more space in the room. But they also shared that, ultimately, owning their space felt both promising and powerful. We connected the movement experience to the parallel process experienced in Mac's life within their community, family, and world. Mac recognized how they could incorporate and embody a more present, aligned, and open stance in relational interactions.

In the next session, Mac told me they had honored the embodied work and felt safe sharing their identity, coming out to their father and grandparents during a family dinner. Mac continued to process the essential work ahead and the patience required to support their family to receive their truth. Each session created a ritual: To begin with movement and embrace the genuine connection to Mac's outer experiences and inner desires.

Vignette 15 Intervention: Honoring Space

Activity Prompt: Explore the following prompt within the clinical session: Notice the space around you. Explore moving around the room. The provider will model how to stay still and explore crawling, low on the ground, being small, and then explore being tall and taking up space with all body parts. Observe the way both of your bodies move in the room. Play around with making different shapes, stretching, and moving in different directions.

Provider Note: Depending on your therapy setting and the physical space in the room – you as the provider can take this activity outside into nature and explore different times in sessions using different locations such as the office, school, or the child's home. Discuss together the observations and needs the child may feel depending on how they move in various locations.

Chapter 5

Therapeutic Lens Explored
Everyday Life With Kids

The vignettes included in Chapter 4 demonstrate the effects of movement-based psychotherapy and its impacts on sibling and family dynamics. They further illuminate an embodied lens for understanding behavior as movement and challenges as adaptive responses related to individual differences and self-identities. Sibling dynamics and family relationships can foster healthy attachment patterns, meaningful learning, and whole development. They are a microcosm of the global dynamics that occur in our society, which we can observe, practice, and repair for more trusting, integrative, and functional processes within the therapeutic relationship and for the overall support of the parent, family, and child. As a philosopher, writer, author, and spiritual figure, Krishnamurti says, "All life is movement in relationships. There is no living thing on Earth that is not related to something or other" (Krishnamurti, 2012, p. 79).

Movement is with us from the time of conception throughout a child's development. Early life relationships are the starting framework and provide insight into how a child's learned experiences impact their understanding and mental health. Movement exploration between parents and children can unlock confusion and provide resolution. Clinical research has found that child therapy can only be successful if there is significant change within the parents or family dynamic. In my therapeutic work, the family – specifically, the parent – is always included in the sessions. Regarding confidentiality, we agree it's a "when and how" to share information rather than an isolated or secret pact between therapist and child. Therefore, the child develops communication skills and a deeper connection to parents and family while simultaneously holding the therapist as an advocate and team partner with the family. The therapeutic relationship begins when the family (child/parent) enters the dance/movement therapy session. "When changes occur in the way the family system deals with each other, the movement interplay changes, and then the outward display of behavior changes" (Chaiklin & Wengrower, 2016, p. 127).

DOI: 10.4324/9781003363491-6

Goodness of Fit

Therapeutic support with movement can be powerful for children who are unable to verbally communicate about uncomfortable topics and fears. Winnicott focused on examining how mental events in the child's environment affect the child's mind. Winnicott believed, too, in the relationship between parents and the therapist (Gvion & Bar, 2014; Winnicott, 1963).

In the *Journal of Psychotherapy*, researchers referenced Winnicott and the importance of allowing the child/individual to maintain their sense of self, especially when it comes to the parent and child relationship. As described here, "Winnicott (1963) addressed the core in the self that is incommunicado (silent). This part is hidden and encapsulates the person's individuality, and it should be left to stay unfound" (Gvion & Bar, 2014, p. 63). That is to say, it should be honored and given time to emerge during the child's developmental process.

In the *Journal of Psychiatry*, the author describes the longitudinal study done by Chess et al. in New York that became a turning point in mental health, discussing Winnicott's framework of "goodness of fit," which helps assess a child in each environment context. "Transactions between child and parents influenced each other's behavior bidirectionally" (Sravanti, 2017, p. 515; Chess, Thomas, Rutter, & Birch, 1963). Parents play an integral role in their child's optimal development by regulating the child's behavior and providing supportive care. It was also found that when the parents tune into who their child is and are sensitive to their child's temperament, their environment, and their attachment/relationship to the child, the child will gain long-term emotional and health benefits (Sravanti, 2017). "Attunement and mirroring use the whole body or some aspect of the body to follow a child's actions. These are the initial techniques that allow the therapist to learn about the child's personal nonverbal language" (Tortora, 2017, p. 291). In the *Dancing Dialogue*, attunement is defined as "a person's matching of a particular quality of another person's movement, which does not completely depict the entire shape, form, attitude, or rhythmic aspects simultaneously, as occurs in mirroring" (Tortora, 2017, p. 499).

Parents frequently observe and recognize individual differences, whether it's in their children when comparing one sibling to another within the same family or even as they witness changes in their children over time. A key method in working with neurodiverse and twice-exceptional children (as explored in Chapter 3) is the gift of learning how to parent the child in front of you, not the child you imagine (SENG, n.d., 2024). This concept can and needs to be applied to all children. Giving permission to learn, fail, recover, and try again in each moment supports the solidification of learned experiences and strengthens one's fortitude to do more. Therefore, as a child undergoes development, we can examine their movement patterns and establish a foundation for comprehending our own child or the client we are assisting. This foundation should be characterized by acceptance, providing an adaptable space within which growth and setbacks can occur, free from any sense of regret or judgment.

Sibling Dynamics

In working with families, I am still baffled by the number of parents who accept sibling rivalry. Parents tolerate children fighting, and the animosity further develops. But with years of sibling work, I believe and experience sibling connection as a marker for how we relate within our friendships, communities, and future relationships (Allemand, Steiger, & Fend, 2015). A sibling is a live-in model for practicing emotional regulation, shared attention, problem-solving, and collaboration. A sibling is the one person who experiences life in the family home and with the parental unit, sharing memories and life during the same time period, while simultaneously having potentially different perspectives due to their own nature and individual distinctions. The sibling dynamic cements one's understanding, role, and individuation in life. The sibling dynamic, however, does need to be modeled, fostered, and taught. So when parents say it's normal for siblings to be rivals, I encourage a deeper look at why this upset is occurring in the first place. What we experience and foster at home – such virtues as respect, patience, tolerance, curiosity, bravery, cooperation, honor, pride, value, and trust – can be emulated in our decisions and communities for years to come.

It's important to note that the sibling dynamic begins before a child is brought home after being born; how a parent sets up a sibling for the new arrival. In my practice, I encourage parents to acknowledge the importance of decisions not based on the new child in the family but because the older child is ready for that next step. For instance, is the older child getting a "big new bed" because the baby is taking away the crib or because the older child is truly ready for a new bed?

Setting children up for decisions and the "why" of choices helps enable autonomy and omission of blame and guilt. When children are in their early years, toddler siblings become passionate about holding a particular toy, voicing a feeling, or attracting attention. It is helpful to teach children to communicate what is allowed versus what is not, encouraging a child to recognize what his sibling can touch, hold, reach, or communicate. The child says, "You may not hold my Legos, but you may watch me build, hand me the red ones, or you can wait and play with the Legos next." The commonality of the preferred task is the focus here: There are endless options, and the available choices allow for receptive and cooperative play. When two children argue over a toy, the focus is not on taking away the item but instead acknowledging the shared goal, that the children admire and crave the same idea, token, or toy. When siblings learn at an early age that they have commonalities, that they have choices, and that they both/all have time and space, the sibling dynamic is bonded and blossoms.

Clinical Integration of DMT

The timing of interactions (parental responses such as impatience or indulgence) and the space (the physical environment and proximity between parent and child) impact the communication and connections built upon in a therapeutic setting and throughout a child's daily life. The dance/movement therapy lens allows for integrative embodied practice between siblings and a way for communication to be understood and fostered. The developing child needs to feel valued within his/her/their family and that they are not a burden within the parental and family dynamic. Supporting siblings to collaborate, appreciate one another's differences, and use connection further promotes independence and respect (Bretherton, Fritz, Zahn-Waxler, & Ridgeway, 1986). Mutual respect enables siblings to see one another's strengths and seek one another out for support and help.

When working with siblings and the family system, the technique of using opposites is a helpful tool to spark creativity and connection. Since accessing creative and interactive approaches may be met with reluctance by parents and providers, using opposites brings simplicity and a clear directive to the desired goal. For instance, when approaching a psychological concept with the child, you, the provider, can acknowledge the physical state in the interaction (i.e., sitting posture, quickened speed) and then explore the opposite, such as standing up, moving slower, thinking slower, etc. (further examples were shared in Chapter 4, Vignette 4). By accessing variations and our options with the child, we can better notice reservations, holdings, patterns, and the potential for flexible adaptive learning.

Notice the body stance of the child during all verbal dialogue, be aware of patterns in how the child sits, visually examines the room, or shifts posturally within the therapeutic environment. Providers can explore sibling dynamics through postural changes and attention. When we look at how a child enters a room, from the held posture of the shoulders to the neck tilt and the patterning resemblance between family members, we gain insight into familial relationships and the internal state of the individual. In addition, thinking about how our facial affect communicates and models a sense of connection or distance sheds light on the importance of facial recognition and attention. Furthermore, facial affect and emotional states of the body within embodied recognition can support one's perceptions of the internal body and signal messages of ease or, conversely, anxiety. Again, paying attention to the body's subtle and meaningful patterning supports overall well-being and connection. How the individual stands in a room, greets others, or physically moves toward or away from a stimulus (i.e., a test, a peer, a parent) supports the importance of body-based awareness, interventions, and what I call body knowledge.

Children are experts in all ways of moving and they demonstrably communicate using the body. When an adult, care provider, or educator understands how to observe, meet and expand on a child's movement repertoire with an expansive and flexible movement vocabulary, the child develops a more relaxed and adaptive way of responding to various stimuli and environments. A child having a tantrum has a short range of chaotic movements; a child with rigidity is restricted and hinders movement. But children who are highly adaptable in their ideas/mindset are equally more agile and able to move and respond adequately to the presented situation. Therefore, what we see in the body's movements is a parallel process to the psychological, mental, and emotional state. This "tell-all" is critical to supporting health and fostering relationships between children and parents, peers, and siblings. These movements and body states are experienced throughout a child's daily interactions, and in this way, the child's surroundings are influenced by the internal (self) and external (other).

Since movement exists in relation to a child's world, awareness of the environment that siblings and families occupy is a prerequisite for understanding family dynamics and should be used during the therapeutic process. The home environment depicts the throughline in which the family exchanges meaningful, often familiar, yet disruptive patterns. Noticing the vantage point of each child creates a lens and perspective of that child's experience and for further treatment protocols. From one child's point of view, territory is defined by the materials that occupy an area and to whom they belong. Noticing that a sibling may have more of a "monopoly" may indicate that child's status or role. Another child may feel strongly about their territory's colors, sounds, or temperature. With the therapeutic focus on the home, community, and school environment, we are attuned to setting up the child for successful, meaningful growth and learning throughout their daily interactions. With siblings, we can have them share what they observe, and explore what they notice about the structure of their home and how that environment came to be.

Children with limited words may benefit from picture cards featuring images and written words that indicate a toy area, and building higher-elevation storage spaces can invite communication with a parent when requesting an item. Creating space within a room to provide for sensory breaks, check-ins, and personal belongings is also beneficial. Children need to feel they are not an inconvenience and have a purpose in a well-organized environment, and the thoughtfully designed areas in a home and parental understanding of a child's perspective facilitate this value. Again, when possible, offering therapeutic interactions, observations, or feedback within the home environment provides a throughline within treatment to best support the whole child – mind, body, and spirit.

Everyday Life

Additionally, each child has a role within the family system. Inviting therapeutic dialogue and body-based practices creates meaning for truly inhabiting these roles and being aware of the essential needs of one to the other. An example of creating a family structure with the body is to have a child mold their family into postures, poses, and the facial affect that indicate his/her/their role in the family and relation to one another. This intervention enables embodied awareness from that child's perspective and invites parents to notice how a child perceives their role and family system. By participating in this activity, families exploring the visual and motoric representation of their system start to reveal patterns, relational tensions, and connections within moments. These movement experientials invite instant feedback, open discussion, and intrinsic, sensed changes for the betterment of the family unit.

I have witnessed the stunned expressions of parents who observe their family dynamics before their very eyes and embrace their children in a way that is novel and celebrated. I have witnessed children situating parents back-to-back, across the room, and even over the children. A child may also appear in the imagery of movement as a spec within the family portrait, an enmeshed attachment of a single parent, or in refusal of a sibling. All the options of family dynamics are felt within the movement-based depiction while also providing an opportunity for pivoting, shifting, replacing, evolving, and safely moving through the family system with ease, as opposed to what may unfold upon merely speaking about such dynamic perspectives. With movement opportunities, there seems to be a reduction of blame and a more expansive space for curiosity and play. The child gains resolve when the family witnesses an embodied display of feelings and emotional exchanges within the therapeutic setting.

Vignettes Explored

In "Kaleidoscope Play" (Chapter 4, Vignette 2), children can find commonality, understanding, and acceptance in their body state and movement choices, bringing together an inclusive mindset and omitting isolation and despair. Movement in the body and observing the child's physicality in relation to his/her/their emotional needs allows for the attunement originally intended in our relational existence.

> Knowledge, or K, according to Bion (1962), is the inner willingness to be in real emotional contact with oneself and others: "in other words, to be in a K state of mind involves the emotional ability to carry the connection with others without possessiveness, to be in an emotional and intimate connection, but without totality and exclusivity."
> (Gvion & Bar, 2014, pp. 62–63; Bion, 1962)

When control or a power dynamic exists between children, the children are isolated, labeled, and separated from one another. Societal labels identify a child as "bossy, rude, fresh, a jerk, etc.," but such immediate adult judgments give little forethought to the child's perspective or internal dysregulation/need. With added insight, we can better understand the child's need for control and safety, which, in this case, is exhibited by asserting one's own organization over another. When a child shows this raw and real contact, and we slow down, omit labels, and seek perspective in looking at the child's body as controlling or being controlled, each child can connect to the other in a shared agreement to find safety and trust. In these moments, which may seem maladaptive, the need to take over, or even the adult's need to separate children, are familiar patterns. Instead of repeating this familiar response, I encourage providers, parents, and children to develop the ability to step into the less familiar. This more adaptive response fosters inclusive movement to rearrange the interaction, building communication and acceptance with one another.

Synaptic Movement and Our Bodies Moving

As described in Chapter 2, therapeutic lens discussion, we look at the planes of movement to support the child to move in a horizontal pattern, parallel to one another to join in completing the desired task, each organized and coexisting instead of over, above, or separate from the other. The horizontal pattern shows up repeatedly in our interactions and within the structure of the body (Groff, 1995). A sort of playful push and pull, or dance, occurs.

When we look at mitochondria, the cell's energy centers, we see a horizontal pattern of synaptic movement from left to right. This synaptic movement is associated with eAPT intake, a process that occurs in every cell and affects energy levels by transferring molecules across cells. This process helps to create and support strength, body mass, and energy levels and can even reduce fatigue (Wang, Li, Qian, et al., 2017). This regulatory action is a critical starting point for all integrative methods: the horizontal plane. Again and again, movement expresses our biological makeup and predisposition toward health. Movement expression connects within the body, external interactions, and relationships to mimic and produce adaptive patterns that support the unity needed for health and connection (Koopman, Beyrath, Fung, et al., 2016). This dimension of movement allows for a softening to arise, a new sense of safety from coexisting and collaborating in the space of acceptance and slowing down the goal for a process-oriented state of being. The horizontal plane is the dimension in which we move within a side-to-side pattern, with the emphasis being more side to side than the front and back (in dance/movement therapy, we equate this to a tabletop image). The side-to-side motion is reminiscent of the connections in rocking, swaying, and holding a loved one. The horizontal plane provides a safe parallel connection, and a foundational space. To better understand the planes of movement, you can read in "Transform a Child in Your Life" (Chapter Four, Vignette 5), about the three-dimensional planes and the analogy of the child and the castle.

But what happens when a child is moving separately from others and has not been noticed or reflected on by another? Subtle movement often goes unobserved, which can be more harmful than we realize. In "The Movement Experiment" (Chapter Four, Vignette 3), you can see the imminent danger created when we fail to notice the body and ignore or laugh at our children's movements. Therapy is limited and potentially maladaptive when only words are treated as the highest focus. During the therapeutic session, we cannot disregard the physical movements and needs present in every moment through a child's bodily interactions and movement profiles.

The child's movement profile supports the clinical understanding of the body's presentation and how the body's movement parallels the emotional and psychological needs supported in therapeutic sessions. The movement profile establishes effort qualities (the intentions of a child's movements, use of weight, space, time, and flow) and the individual's postures (shape); facial affect (expressions); dimensional ways of relating to their own body, others, and their environment; and the use of sensory intake/processing. By identifying individual movement patterns and what I call the "true temperature check," we get a baseline for and fuller view of the child's emotional regulation and co-occurring needs. The temperature check is not only what we do with a thermometer to identify a fever; it is also how we know our child's movement profile, demeanor, and patterns of interaction (mind, body, and spirit). When a parent is supported to recognize the child's body posturing, timing (speed of the voice, walking, transitioning, playing), and experience of his/her/their body in relationship to the world (i.e., awareness of having a spot of food on their face, having to use the toilet, taking a helping of food, or sitting in a loving or even terrifying exchange of emotions), they have an embodied experience of their child. The three areas of embodied experience are mental temperature (assess whether the child is running "hot or cold" by noticing language, voice tone, and particular phrasing), body temperature (assess whether the child is receptive or dismissive by noticing posture, facial affect, and gestures), and soul temperature (assess whether the child is filled with life or depleted by noticing energy level, vibrancy, and felt sense).

Patterns and Connections

The body holds information in the reception of or withdrawal from fear/danger. Knowing the child's patterns brings further insight into when there is a drastic or even a subtle shift. Have you noticed if the child came into the session with a pep in their step, had their head slumped-over, or a racing tone of voice? How a child moves and demonstrates awareness of his/her/their body and its impact on others is critical to social-emotional learning and overall health. Without this temperature awareness, we miss crucial cues from a child in need. When I think of the hostile and tragic events imparted by children onto others, such as the enormity of gun violence in schools over the past decade, I consider the following questions: Who sees the child when they wake up? Who did the child see as they walked down the street, through the door, and into the school room?

The body holds emotional experiences and releases feelings through heartful and harmful movements (Van Der Kolk, 2014). Acknowledging the body through our lens of communication, education, and health, we allow for opportunities to prevent danger and increase safety for one another and all our children. In my lectures on mindful teaching for the moving child, educators are informed of the motion patterns of children and their awareness of body movements, postures, facial affect, and the important interplay between our bodies during the educational day. The insights that come with studying the body enable increased meaningful learning within the classroom, safe interactions between teachers and students in the educational environment, and information for continued academic growth and overall well-being. Again, in teaching using a dance/movement therapy lens to understand the body and how experiences are felt and organized through movement, critical communication is also taught.

The vignettes in Chapter 4 explore some therapeutic sessions during the holiday season and within the common dynamics throughout the calendar year. By looking at patterns and acknowledging the individual child's processes over the course of a family history, the family can be guided to accept and move toward prior planning, present communication, and successful interactions. Periods outside of school during holidays and throughout the calendar year will bring perspective to our children's emotional regulatory needs and ever-evolving patterns. Within the therapeutic practice, providers may experience an influx and a consecutive decline in services throughout any academic year. These ebbs and flows of clinical practice shed light on the collective consciousness present in our society and the heightened impacts of societal demands and seasonal changes. Family dynamics often arise most clearly during holidays and other social interactions with family members.

Supporting parents and families during these holiday transition times may bring further connection and ease to the child and parent relationship. For instance, as explored in "The Three Ps for a Peaceful Holiday" (Chapter Four, Vignette 8), allowing the parent to acknowledge the three Ps – pruning, preferences, and practicing can be extremely effective during the holiday season (see Figure 5.1). The three Ps can be applied without limitation to other heightened states of social gathering and cultural ritual states. Here, I will elaborate on my three Ps concept.

Pruning, noticing what happened in the past after a sensory embodied awareness, such as how lights, sounds, and other aspects of an environment elicit ease or discomfort, is the first P. How did space in a room invite

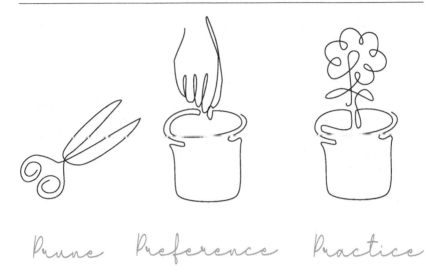

Prune   Preference   Practice

Figure 5.1 The 3 Ps

closeness or isolation? With these embodied observations and reflections, the individual is then able to access alternatives to use in their current family dynamic with their own children. We invite the family to prepare themselves by acknowledging feelings, "shoulds," and "mantras" typically heard during these heightened occasions.

Preferences is the second P. In these activities, the family explores sensory and body-based needs. Identifying the individual differences of each family member supports a deeper understanding and effective follow through for engaging in the event interactions. Additionally, identifying any needed changes to the physical space, the child's need for breaks, or any assignments necessary for carrying out in the here and now occur during preferred activities.

Practicing, lastly, allows a family to try on methods before a large event (i.e., birthday, holiday, special meal). Practicing is always an invitation to move, observe, and play with ideas to enable joint attention, communication, problem-solving, and creative exploration. Noticing the preferences and perspectives of family members plus self-reflection promotes opportunities for enacting positive change and embracing preferred states of being. Now a clear plan can manifest for each relational exchange.

Expectations and Common Dynamics

A common question in family dynamics arises around household chores, tasks, and expectations; how to motivate children and, more so, how to get compliance. Joining children in the practice of daily living skills, sharing in brushing teeth, tidying a space, and finding a connection to meaningfully placed objects in a house can help create a sense of belonging in the environment and value in the family system (Villines, 2021). Chores become a way of interacting together and playfully moving through the day instead of moments of tension or affliction. There becomes no distinction between chores and life, but rather it is a fluid dance from one room to the next; objects, clothes, and food are connected and used, organized, exchanged, expanded on, and then returned to be explored another time. The exchange creates an opportunity for children to see a continuous working through and creative art form within each interaction and that even washing a dish or picking up a toy holds purpose and value in a family system.

When a parent identifies noncompliance, I typically acknowledge the child's lack of meaningful connection to that task. For example, the child may not understand why or how the concept works within the relationship with objects or parents. When there is meaning and a social connection (i.e., this is a task shared with a parent or because of an intrinsic understanding), compliance occurs regularly. At times, the why may not serve the individual child, as when using silverware to pick up food may, at a young age, not serve the same purpose of getting food into the mouth, chewing, and swallowing. The child may notice that he/she/they could do so easier with hands and in a speedier, more functional way, so the meaning of using silverware has less merit. In these instances, we lean on etiquette and social norms to teach and help the child register that the task is for the other and not solely for the self. We use silverware for the purposes of etiquette, to keep our hands clean, and to elicit a civilized manner.

When we separate meaning, function, and etiquette, there is less opportunity for upset and frustration. The therapeutic exchange can again model and sort out what compliance with a task means and provide strategies to relate to and support family interactions. Making this distinction is imperative before any behavioral modification or task teaching, as it creates meaning and, more so, an acknowledgment of the child's inner experience and rightful response to the expectation. In this way, credit is given to the child, and when we value a child's understanding, we open channels for more receptivity, opportunity, and trust.

Identities and Behaviors

In my professional work, I have explored how identities form from conception and seem to gain traction as the baby develops. Some parents experience their child's identity as being there from the beginning, and others are learning who their child is each day. One of the areas I find helpful is acknowledging a mother's patterns of sleep, cravings, thoughts, and emotional needs during pregnancy and to further explore how these are then re-experienced and relevant to the unborn child's life. When we invite a connection between the journey into the world and how the child moves through childhood, we learn valuable information that enables the child to be accepted and seen for who they have been all along. This acceptance evokes a sense of relief, learning, and a bit of humor in daily life.

Additionally, how the child enters the world is the initial indication of their coping and adaptive responses to the sensory world. How that child accommodates and habituates to his/her/their surroundings can impact the experience of the relationships and environments in their daily experiences. These early life phases are just one of many factors that contribute to the individual child's overall essence and further growth. We seek not to place blame or try and cipher out each cause but rather to use this as a knowledge-based approach for understanding how much we already know about our children. I use the metaphor of a pool of water (see Figure 5.2) to support the impact that parents and care providers have on children: Each drop of water is a variable placed before and experienced by the child – the family history, trauma, environment, parental dynamic, educational system, medical background, etc. We can't sift the water to determine which variable caused what in and of the child, but we can certainly know the child is in that pool of variables/influences and we can support the child to swim and not to sink. The pool analogy invites an awareness of the many factors that impact a child's developmental differences and relationships while also negating blame and parental despair. This allows parents to feel empowered in an active role in their child's development and to find joy and resilience in teaching the child how to swim.

Our goal as providers and parents is to help children find safety within their developmental story and support them through what they find threatening. In clinical diagnosis, we look at a child's behaviors and symptoms based on criteria that measure the length of time, frequency, and duration. The child's outwardly displayed behaviors are measured against other children in the same developmental age range. Consequently, expectations of the child based on age and environment have a strong connection to what the provider determines are diagnostic indicators for clinical care and focus. For

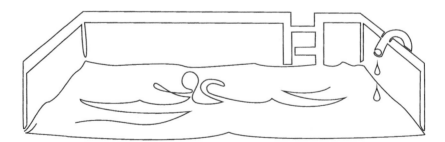

Figure 5.2 The Pool Analogy

instance, from birth to about three years old, a child's deficits and strengths may exist in their ability to respond to the sensory world. The infant and toddler work to respond to sights, sounds, temperatures, and tastes. When a child struggles to regulate their senses, we see a challenge and a diagnosis may follow. Next, the four- to six-year-old is thrust into the world of others, places, and spaces, including play dates, attending preschool, and social expectations. From these ages, providers look beyond the senses to assess a child's diagnosis, evaluating their response to transitions, separation, and emotional regulation. We expect children to be able to move through the world with others and transition successfully. Moving on, when seven- to nine-year-olds are given orders to sit, listen, and respond, attention becomes the highest priority in these age groups. Adults' expectations of increasing the child's capacity to focus and the ability to discern where, when, and how to respond become of the utmost importance. Then, at age ten to thirteen, as adolescents reap the impact of those early stages of existence, experiencing and recovering from sensory system overload (i.e., living in the same body, experiencing the same input/feedback year after year but with developing body parts), using tools, navigating social pressures, norms, and academic expectations, and world awareness may result in anxiety, pain, and depression, as identified in Chapter one. Thus, we see that with each expectation, a child's display of emotions and physical behaviors or movements takes on a new shape. When we witness the movements of the child as predictable and in relation to their world experience throughout their development, life feels much more manageable. The child is a full "being" experiencing life with mind, body, and spirit.

Honoring Individual Differences and Understanding Identity

To honor individual differences and understand identity, we need to push toward accepting these senses and feeling states. As human beings, the word "being" is unique to our species in that it's a verb, an action that takes form based on the senses, feelings, and movements we live with and in everyday life. When we hear about mental illness, we often hear statistics on suicide, medication, addiction, and overdose (alcoholism, technology, sugar intake, etc.). The focus of treatment may be to stop the feeling state, control the pain, and isolate the problem. But to do that makes us inhuman – robotic, nonfeeling. "Being" is actually living within our feelings and accepting that the alternative is not to exist. Feelings invite information we can learn to harness and use for growth and understanding, compassion, and empathy (especially for ourselves and for the child). I hope this book can instill the insights needed to prove that embodiment – truly experiencing feelings in the body through movement or internal expression delivered externally – matters and that since we are "moving" through childhood, we must help our children celebrate this dance.

A major tenet of individual identity includes gender labels, the definition of which now includes boy, girl, and nonbinary. Gender refers to socially constructed norms, behaviors, and roles within society, and research looks to identify gender-related patterns to support interventions and relational needs. The use of movement within therapeutic exchanges allows for an inclusive paradigm that supports verbal skills and the visual-spatial components indicative of learning across different gender identities (Gurian, 2010). Using the dance/movement therapy lens to view the body and movement places importance on the child's individual profile while being accurate about what we witness in the interactions and exchanges with and by the child. This fully accepting therapy method stays true to understanding and fostering the whole child, no matter the identity or unique qualities being presented or developed while supporting the exploration and validation the child seeks.

As we saw in "Honoring Space" (Chapter 4, Vignette 15), I match, mirror, and attune to the child's preferred way of being, stance, and identity. By creating a trusting relationship within the embodied practices of dance/movement therapy, the child develops trust and self-respect. A study done by the *American Journal of Dance Therapy* explored "the actions and attitudes regarding LGBTQI and gender-nonconforming communities" and found that "for dance/movement therapists, one's awareness must extend to personal movement patterns and how they relate to behaviors, thoughts, feelings, and aesthetic choices," and "how personal movement preferences and sociocultural background influence all domains of treatment, including aesthetic choices and the observation, assessment, and analysis of movement" (Kawano, Cruz, & Tan, 2018, p. 19). The clinical provider must continuously work to identify their own movement patterns and biases to provide the utmost safety and support to the full identity presented by each child. The interplay between therapist and child is a beautiful, constant dance in which a felt experience (transference/countertransference) is recognized in the body and processed with respect and acceptance of the child's individual profile and needs.

Areas for Diagnostic Assessment

Related to identity, I encourage you to look at the body as a guide into the deep internalization of psychological and emotional states. As the child walks into the space, from the waking moments to the sleeping state, the body holds a parallel process to what is being felt. I have found ten observational areas that can be used in evaluating and, more importantly, bring insight for treatment interventions (see Figure 5.3).

The ten areas, as diagrammed in Figure 5.3, provide the baseline temperature of the child and more clinical indication for your treatment or work with siblings/children. By studying these areas, as I will further

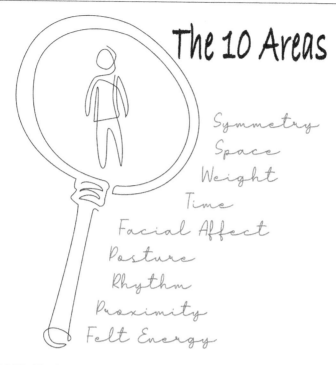

The 10 Areas

Symmetry
Space
Weight
Time
Facial Affect
Posture
Rhythm
Proximity
Felt Energy

Figure 5.3 The Ten Areas

explain, during your intake process and additional clinical care, you can get a true read of the child's given state and mental health needs. Look at a child's **symmetry** (1): How their head sits, shoulder elevation/constriction, mouth/tongue posture, and frame, particularly with a sitting posture (i.e., in a "W"). Be aware of any asymmetry in the bodies of children with pathology, illness, or even just simple weakness. Asymmetry can be more than just a slightly bigger foot or a raised eyebrow. It can be more obvious, such as a child's head tilting prominently to one side or favoring one side of their body when walking. Other examples include a stiff-legged walk with a relaxed upper body, as if the arms and legs are disconnected, or one eye converging toward the center of the face while the other eye remains focused straight ahead. There are many ways that asymmetry can manifest in the body, both in posture and in movement expression. The qualities of **space** (2), **weight** (3), and **time** (4) indicate how a child moves through the environment and particular kinesthetic space, the intentionality of weightiness in the body, and the frequency or speed in which he/she/they move. These concepts are rooted in the LBMA (Laban Bartenieff Movement Analysis) field of work, in which movement has been described, visualized, and interpreted in order to document the commonalities and throughlines of movement within and between bodies (Laban, 1960). The studies of body movement extend into what is called BESS (body, effort, shape, space). Imagine understanding how each aspect of our movement holds meaningful insight into our dynamic relationships, spatial harmony, and psycho-emotional integration.

Kinesthetic space (2) is the perceived boundary between the physical body (where the body [the skin/bone] is located) and the surrounding "negative" space, which is the area around the body where a child moves and navigates. It is within this space that a child's awareness of these two dimensions is actively engaged and manipulated. This phenomenon becomes evident when we observe how a child instinctively draw their focus inward to their body to maintain balance, such as when walking on a tightrope or simply navigating everyday life with both feet on the ground. Conversely, we can also witness children who resemble whirling dervishes, effortlessly enveloping their surroundings as they move through their environment, not seemingly connected to their actual bodies' whereabouts.

This concept parallels our observations of a child's connection to their core, breath, and body versus their awareness of their limbs. Among the various inquiries we can pose, we might wonder whether a child frequently bumps their arms while walking through school or if they exhibit signs of being clingy or overly reliant on walls for stability and tracking.

The analysis of movement holds great significance and serves as an invaluable perspective through which to explore the realms of psychology and mental health care. By doing so, we can not only understand but also replicate and infuse meaning into every interpersonal exchange between individuals, particularly in the context of the interactions between ourselves and our children, which are pivotal in therapeutic settings.

Weight (3) as indicated throughout the book, is represented by a child's strong/heavy qualities as opposed to the lighter movements and expressions of the body. Weightedness and the use of this quality can be an indication of what is typically seen as a child seeming grounded or not. Whereas time (4) indicates the elements of quick and sustained movements that are expressed across interactions and experienced within the child's body. The qualities of space, weight, and time, first discussed in Chapter 2, will continue to be explored in Chapter 6. The movement analysis is extensive and a much needed lens to infiltrate the field of psychology and mental health care – only to emulate and bring meaningfulness to each body-to-body exchange, the lived experiences, and interactions between us and our children are critical in therapeutic exchange.

The child's **facial affect** (5) indicates the congruence or incongruence between emotions and physical presence or the range of expressiveness versus decline and disassociation. A child's **posture** (6) may be indicative of the family and school/community environment and genetic patterns and may reveal a metaphorical emotional burden carried on the shoulders. The rhythm (7) of a child's interactions shed further light on their ability to find ease and flow in connections or a staccato, jarring, rigid misalignment. Initiation (8) is another interesting element of observation: To identify how a child leads and controls the interactions and emotional exchange versus being controlled or disconnected from others; identifying how a child presents ideation, intent, and activation; or joins and expands on ideas, function, and movement. This leads to assessing a child's ability to repeat, learn, and mimic.

The last two areas are observational and interpreted by the provider. The **proximity** (9) to the therapist, between parent and child, and child and the physical environment or even his/her/their body (how a child holds their own hands or feet) adds additional insight to relational dynamics and individual developmental needs. Lastly, the **felt energy** (10) of a child – whimsy or reserve, high-spirited or withdrawn, presence in the room or distance, as from another universe – can be experienced in any interaction and create a relevant measurement of the psychological and emotional underpinning of the child's daily life and relational self.

Patterns and Building Relationships

As the provider, we model how to communicate by narrating what is happening around the child, using sights, sounds, textures, tastes, and smells. We invite the child to notice and sometimes, more so, the adult to join the child in noticing what is being felt in and around the body. This technique is also useful in eliciting motivation and grit.

Carol Dweck's work emphasizes the growth-mindset approach to acknowledging processes instead of the outcome or dichotomy of good versus bad (Dweck, 2006). When we tell a child what we see, this invites increased communication and exploration of bewilderment, internal processing, and self-compassion. For an emotional-themed example, imagine the child is crying: Instead of saying, "You are sad," we can say, "I see your tears, your face looking down." The child then gets to decipher their true state; they can adjust or stay in this emotional release. While learning emotional labels/language can bring meaningful information into relational communication, in the child/adult dynamic the labeling may elevate the labeled feeling, may be misidentified and can even create a power dynamic. For instance, I have witnessed countless stories of parents sharing how their child seemed sad, was told he was sad, and then used this type of dynamic in a way that seemed to gain the child a reward, such as a dessert or more time delaying the challenging task. When we instead observe the child's positioning, it is the child who is allowed to be sad or to just use the release of tears; and in their own awareness, they are able to adjust.

For a functional example, imagine the child has drawn a picture: The parent says, "I see the color purple and the use of large brushstrokes," thus enabling the child to communicate their own intent intrinsically and intentionally for the drawing without being swayed by the parent's choice of label or pressure to produce a particular performance/product. The child further develops his/her/their sense of self-identity and personal truths. The parent becomes a partner in truth-telling, identifying what is there, omitting judgments and misconceptions, encouraging the child to experience authenticity and what it means to be a truth-teller. A helpful tool in therapeutic work with parent and child is to support observational skills (having the parent notice how their child moves in addition to the parent's perception of the child's feelings) and accuracy of communication (saying how the child moves, sounds, etc., instead of the assumed emotion). Some key areas for exploring observation and accuracy can be during transitions, meals, toileting routines, as well as with sleep and eating patterns. These critical parts of a child's daily life involve not only big feelings but significant movement patterns. These areas are key markers of the child's ever-evolving autonomy and separation. When we look at a baby's sleep patterns while assessing a distinct correlation to their sensory needs and developing body, the interventions become clear. A child doesn't become a poor sleeper or avoid sleep to be difficult or because sleep isn't needed anymore (which a toddler's parents may say if the child stops napping); rather, the way a child comes into their ability to recoup and repair evolves and changes with their growing interests, social-emotional demands, and sensory system.

Sensory and Body-Based Needs

As the child develops, it's important to consider their sensory system and body-based needs. Identifying soothing patterns for the child provides the necessary intervention tools for successful sleep and daily living skills throughout their development. Again, the child isn't a bad sleeper; they just need to fall asleep differently now than they have before. A baby rocked to sleep in the dark may now need to be given visual input to release their system from the day's overload and transition to closing their eyes. There are many examples here, with the main emphasis being (1) learn the child's present habits for soothing; (2) be open to adapting the process as the child evolves; (3) return to familiar patterns should the child become stuck; and, when in doubt, remember to observe the child's movement patterns to find ways to join the child where they are instead of giving up. Being a detective within the child's life brings meaningful connection to the developmental years. This ability to read the body's cues and adapt to what is needed fosters nuance, intentionality, creativity, and optimism in parenting and the clinical care of the child/client.

The brilliance of the dance/movement therapy approach and using an integrative lens for working with children is that activation occurs over theory. Growth happens when a child moves from thinking and identify-ing into actual internalization, which occurs viscerally at the body level. For instance, as a child sorts through the features of his/her/their iden-tity, exploration can arise through curiosity or, sometimes, a destructive, controlling, and even abrasive manner. In these moments, if we identify the growth, we invite exploration of the unknown for the child, and in instances of aggression, supporting them to consider lowering the dial on the intensity. This is more supportive and applicable than asking a child to stop or admonishing them to be ashamed of their individual journey. Some examples from the vignettes from Chapter 4 show work on shrinking and growing within the body. This physical exploration invites an embodied, felt experience of the growing pattern. Additionally, the energy extended beyond the confines of our physical body – distinguishing between the boundaries of our body and the surrounding space (often referred to as negative space) – serves as a means for individuals to better connect with their core. This connection offers them the opportunity to draw inward or seek refuge as necessary, guided by a sense of comfort and self-care, rather than as a retreat driven by harm or shame.

When working with parents and educators, I also encourage the tech-nique of turning down the dial to create opportunities and a sense of mod-eration in interactions between adults and children (see Figure 5.4 Turning the Dial). This shift away from "all or nothing" provides yet another exam-ple of flexible thinking and adaptation. When we think about challenges that come from observing a child's identity and present behaviors, resilience is best created through opportunities for change and exploration within the body. Each time our body lifts a heavy weight, our muscles develop not because of the frequency with which we lift the weight, but rather because the body adapts and expands to meet the needs of the load and survive in a new space. Imagine if we took every chance to build resilience, how the judgments and expectations would fall aside and how we could reside in the acceptance of what is happening in the body. To truly see what is in front of us and allow for ever-evolving growth and opportunity, it is imperative that we see behaviors as movement and strip away restrictive labels.

Outside of a fixed state or a labeled feeling, the child's actions are bet-ter seen, supported, and joined. The child moves in a particular direc-tion, with a quality, and intention to connect and learn. This experience is ever-changing and adaptive. When we say what we see in front of us, instead of using labels, the body of the child is able to connect to his/her/their truth and make changes or sit within the feeling state. This is the therapeutic alliance: Fostering the ability to sit in the unknown and dis-comfort, if it arises, and to see how it serves the individual. This is how feelings are moved from one moment to the next, not via an identifying diagnosis or label.

Turning the dial

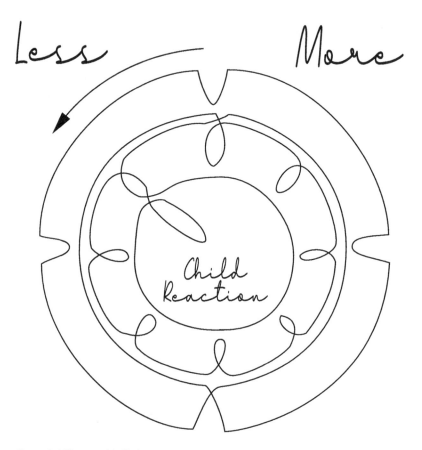

Less   More

Child Reaction

Figure 5.4 Turning the Dial

In my dance/movement therapy sessions, I explore postural changes as they relate to the emotional and physical relationship to the other (person or environment). The postural changes can be seen in a child's shaping of their body (are they hunched over, straight, or curving their body) or the flow of the body (does the child move seamlessly in attunement to our conversation or seem stuck or detached). The beauty I find in dance/movement therapy is that movement may represent different states and feelings for each child, while the child will maintain clear patterns of how he/she/they interact and move in the world.

For some children, flow is related to the ease or resistance felt in moments of communication or connection. On one side, calm/alert flow of movement can be shown in a child comfortably riding a bike, moving through a task with passion, or even writing down ideas in a stream of consciousness. On the flip side is the tension and resistance, as in pushback from a child or the appropriate use of a tight hold for the sake of security, such as holding a hand firmly to cross the street or pulling together to avoid a crash. Applying these concepts brings, yet again, a lens of understanding and purpose to all of our myriad movement tools.

Moderation

Moderation is another component of health that we strive for and support in order to remove extremes and absolutes. I advocate for providers to become team members with families, to avoid telling them what they are doing wrong, and instead to celebrate what works well within that family dynamic, while providing alternatives and psychoeducation when experiences prove to be otherwise maladaptive. Moderation results from looking at the child's capabilities and supporting a range of skills: A child who can sleep independently in their room ultimately gets more opportunities for sleepover experiences with parents, siblings, and friends; a child who can turn off the TV or other technology upon request gets more opportunities for screen time. Self-sufficient, consistent execution by the child not only prompts more expectations in the adult, but also creates opportunities to identify more skills and support more possibilities. We strive for children who have a broad range of skills and a versatile tool kit for coping with and adjusting to their daily needs, who can express their preferences versus insisting "I can't" (i.e., "I prefer to sleep in the same room as my parents tonight," not "I can't sleep alone").

Clinical support can work to strengthen the child's general abilities first and then their ability to choose what is preferred. In the case of preferences, moderation is the difference between expectations and intentions, rules and agreements. When we set intentions, we support an evolving process that brings alignment to the child's purpose and efforts. Conversely, expectations place blame and evoke resistance in a child. Similarly, agreements invite the child and family to set up mutual understanding, while rules evoke feelings of competition, failure, and control. Identifying and mindfully using language that promotes connection and further communication will always support the therapeutic alliance and overall well-being of the child.

In dance/movement therapy, the embodied practice allows the experience to be central in the moment rather than intangibly in the foreground or background. The "law of small things" speaks to the principle of taking each moment at a time (or, in this case, the movement), which brings a connection to the body, validation to the child, and closeness to the relationship/healing process (Brody, 2019). The child's emotional system is not hijacked by external expectations and demands but becomes a meaningful part of developmental growth and necessary transaction. This is the essence of mindfulness at play. In the dance/movement therapy session, the emotional and psychological experiences that occur in the lower limbic regions, ancient systems in the brain, are given room to catch up to current demands. By slowing down and rebuilding through movement, pathways are connected for new positive integration. In our busy lives, the opportunity to sit with, lean in, and slow down in a secure setting, such as the therapeutic space, invites change and healing. With room enough to eventually recognize and bring insight to feeling states, experiences, and relationships, the child can gain perspective and acceptance. Additionally, the family and parent system can offer acceptance and honor the child's adaptive response.

Sharing Control and Transitions

In moments of chaos and dysregulation, children may display a pronounced inclination toward control, attempting to impose order in response to the overwhelming and unfamiliar nature of their experience. In the therapeutic setting, we want to invite opportunities to practice control and model ways a child may put this into action at home, not during states of dysregulation, but rather in the preventative space of priming (before the challenged state) or in regulated moments. Identifying positive aspects of behaviors and traits (that of control or concern) creates opportunities to reveal the adaptive nature of these states and the beneficial qualities that can be applied to a child's developmental schema. The control becomes that of assertiveness and focus for our attunement and understanding. Again, the movement lens fosters a space to not only talk, read, or simply observe these modes of being, but to actually *be* in a state of assertion and awareness: To physically move the body to attain a desired outcome, share an exchange, and feel an intentional connection.

Transitions are often a hot topic in child development, prompting "go to" strategies, articles, and interviews with parents to discuss the difficulties of getting from one place to another. Inevitably, transitions are challenged because of the mere fact that the body has been in a familiar state, and then a gravitational shift takes place to effect moving out of that state and into another. In physics, Newton's law of motion describes a body in motion as keeping the same motion unless acted upon by an outside force. Even the word "force" in the description evokes the pressure involved in the elements at play. It's pretty interesting to consider this as just physics, right? When children act contrary to what is expected, adults may reference these moments as regressions, such occasions when the child has lost their age-appropriate abilities and reverted to an earlier stage of development. This sudden switch in the state is immediately paired with a feeling of discontent and longing, plus fear and exhaustion. A parent or provider may feel as though skills have been lost and a sense of failure ensues. From the child's perspective, though, these moments are referred to as a state of burnout and being overwhelmed, a time of inner restoration and a return to a familiar state. This is the space where learning occurs.

Imagine building a path in the sand. Each time the path is crossed, the grooves deepen and solidify. In this way, a child's regression signals a return to and through a state to regain previously learned skills. To regard these demanding moments as a chance for recuperation from burnout or intense sensory stimulation, as well as a respite from academic pressures, social interactions, and family dynamics, it is advisable to approach the child with an attitude of acceptance and extend an opportunity for them to recover. I encourage caregivers to identify the feeling state these moments elicit, noticing how the exhaustion and point of failure lead to a need to rest and reconnect. Take these inner triggered states and ask,

- If I feel this way, it's possible the child does too.
- How can I support a space for healing and inner ease?
- How might I support the child in this moment while avoiding judgments about what might appear to be a lost skill or a state that will never end?

I find there is profound value in recognizing that what is elicited in us may be just what the child is feeling. They have placed and modeled this state for us to receive, not to guard against or react, but to provide insight and care from a place of understanding and congruence.

Instead of enabling the pattern of an ineffective response in an immediate moment, the provider supports and models a new understanding, which creates a broader opportunity for lasting growth and learning. This requires a big leap in trust that is more easily realized through the felt body and moving interactions with the child, not just with words.

Reactions Versus Responses

Part of understanding identities is how we look at a child's behaviors (movements) in relation to his/her/their environment (persons, place, things, internal systems). By comprehending the difference between behavioral reactions and a child's response to his/her/their sensory system, we can decipher the truth of the child's identity and unlock the child's superpowers. How a child moves through the world in reaction to others (the behavior displayed) is on all fronts an adaptive response to support the child's needs in that particular situation. Some responses are patterned and based on learned experiences, the so-called cause and effect that produced an outcome desirable or needed for that child. However, a behavior has markedly different intentionality than a sensory response, and a behavior results in the specific feeling states of the child (anger, sadness, remorse). Different strategies/responses by the provider/adult can support additional learning and health. For example, a child's intrinsic motivation to get out of a non-preferred task to move on to something more desirable may seem logical (though less desirable by the adult). The child in these situations may make intentional eye contact, repeat the action multiple times (i.e., continue to touch another child's hair) until getting the intended result (to be sent out of the room or separated from the peer) and then express feeling relieved at the outcome, even if reprimanded. Alternatively, a child's adaptive response to survive and move through a sensorily challenged moment will produce a child who maintains minimal to no eye contact, an increased perseveration (inability to stop the challenged response – i.e., making loud sounds and jumping around in the class) and ultimately/consistently result in feeling shame, embarrassment, or guilt. The child in that moment is viewed as the water that spills out of the pitcher that can't be reabsorbed.

The response to each of these situations is different in that a behavioral reaction allows for planning and communication to help the child seek desired outcomes, while increasing the child's ability to take on more novel tasks with scaffolding and support. For sensory responses, the child is best supported by understanding their individual profile before the dysregulation occurs so the child can be provided with empowered options to support survival first, what I call applying the five survival steps (see Figure 5.5): water, food, comfort, collaboration, change in environment, and then options for choosing how to ameliorate the sensory overload. As demonstrated back in Chapter 1, "Shedding Light on Comfort" (Vignette 13) and "The Importance of Being Aware" (Chapter 1, Vignette 16), this is when a child's superpowers – senses that we use every day – come into play. How the child organizes sounds, sights, touch, smell, and taste, as well as the kinesthetic awareness (external processes) and the interception (internal processes), and finally, the body in balance by one's proprioception/vestibular systems contributes to how the child navigates through life. By strengthening our skills to distinguish between behaviors and sensory challenges, we can further elicit the positive momentum needed to support healthy exchange and personal growth for the child. As an optimist, I invite parents and children to accept that they are not a problem to be fixed; they are complex and beautiful beings that we can learn more about and understand deeply.

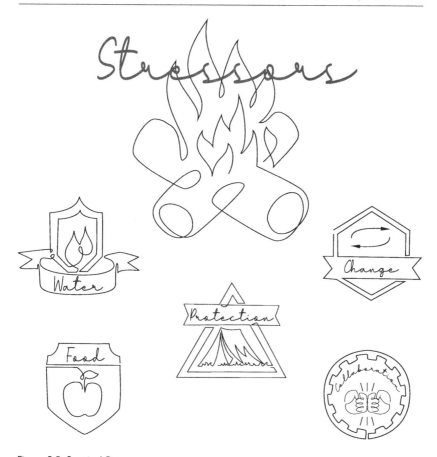

Figure 5.5 Survival Responses

Language (semantics) matters as a conduit between the body and the relational space. I see words as a flowing mechanism between bodies and the grounding element within our wheelhouse of skills. The use of language prompts interpretation and attention to one's thinking and mindset. In the clinical relationship, offering permission to share, speaking with intentionality, and accepting how words impact our exchanges create further understanding of mental health. When we hang only on words, though, we dismiss the body exchange. When we follow only our words we are often left in a predicament of headspace, and when we follow only the body, we may be caught in patterns; but when we follow both the mind and body – not regarding them as separate – we have clear communication and understanding. A simple phrase like "You may move" prompts the child to be in motion, and yet we notice the immediate interpretation of movement, i.e., quickness, jumping, turning, when, in reality, movement can be as simple as a heartbeat, eye flutter, or holding one's posture.

In readings from David Abram's books, *The Spell of the Sensuous*, and *Becoming Animal: An Earthly Cosmology*, I am met with a kindred attunement to the view that all living things and aspects of nature, even the heaviest rock or mountain, has access to movement and interaction with human beings – even the ability to move us into feeling a connection and awareness of our own identity and purpose:

> Although we may be oblivious to the gestural, somatic dimensions of language, having repressed it in favor of strict dictionary definitions and the abstract precision of specialized terminologies, this dimension remains subtly in all our speaking and writing – if that is, our words have any significance whatsoever. For meaning, as we have said, remains rooted in the sensory life of the body. It cannot be completely cut off from the soil of direct, perceptual experience without withering and dying.
>
> (Abram, 2012, p. 80)

We can instill these concepts in the children/clients while working to embody knowledge and self-understanding. The excerpt from "The Discourse of the Birds" (Abstract) says it well, "Other animals, in a constant and mostly unmediated relation with their sensory surroundings, think with the whole of their bodies" (Abram, 2010). We *are* innate movers, not to be ignored or positioned but our expression openly received, shared, and evolved. When we ignore the body and movement, we dull down the senses and avoid the more significant meaning behind what is felt in the body and how this information can provide healing and health. Thankfully, the ability to access emotions and mental health through the body is universal, cross-cultural, socially apt, and physically possible.

References

Abram, D. (2010). The discourse of the birds. *Biosemiotics*, 3(3), 263–275.

Abram, D. (2012). *The spell of the sensuous: Perception and language in a more-than-human world.* Knopf Doubleday Publishing Group.

Allemand, M., Steiger, A. E., & Fend, H. A. (2015). Empathy development in adolescence predicts social competencies in adulthood. *Journal of Personality*, 83(2), 229–241.

Bion, W. R. (1962). The psycho-analytic study of thinking: A theory of thinking. *The International Journal of Psycho-Analysis*, 43, 306–310.

Bretherton, I., Fritz, J., Zahn-Waxler, C., & Ridgeway, D. (1986). Learning to talk about emotions: A functionalist perspective. *Child Development*, 57(3), 529–548.

Brody, S. H. (2019). *The law of small things: Creating a habit of integrity in a culture of mistrust.* National Geographic Books.

Chaiklin, S., & Wengrower, H. (2016). *The art and science of dance/movement therapy: Life is dance, body, movement and dance in psychotherapy* (Vol. 2, pp. 1–351). Routledge Publishing. https://doi.org/10.1080/17432979.2017.1345791

Chess, S., Thomas, A., Rutter, M., & Birch, H. G. (1963). Interaction of temperament and environment in the production of behavioral disturbances in children. *The American Journal of Psychiatry*, 120(2), 142–148.

Dweck, C. S. (2006). *Mindset: The new psychology of success.* Random House Publishing.

Groff, E. (1995). Laban movement analysis: Charting the ineffable domain of human movement. *Journal of Physical Education, Recreation & Dance*, 66(2), 27–30.

Gurian, M. (2010). *Boys and girls learn differently! A guide for teachers and parents.* John Wiley & Sons.

Gvion, Y., & Bar, N. (2014). Sliding doors: Some reflections on the parent–child–therapist triangle in parent work–child psychotherapy. *Journal of Child Psychotherapy*, 40(1), 58–72.

Kawano, T., Cruz, R. F., & Tan, X. (2018). Dance/movement therapists' attitudes and actions regarding LGBTQI and gender nonconforming communities. *American Journal of Dance Therapy*, 40(2), 202–223.

Koopman, W. J., Beyrath, J., Fung, C.-W., Koene, S., Rodenburg, R. J., Willems, P. H., & Smeitink, J. A. (2016). Mitochondrial disorders in children: Toward development of small-molecule treatment strategies. *EMBO Molecular Medicine*, 8(4), 311–327.

Krishnamurti, J. (2012). *Relationships to oneself to others to the world to oneself: To oneself to others to the world to oneself.* Krishnamurti Foundation America.

Laban, R. V. (1960). *The mastery of movement* (First Published Under the Title "Mastery of Movement on the Stage") (2nd Ed., Revised and Enlarged by Lisa Ullmann. [With a Portrait.]). Macdonald & Evans.

SENG. (n.d.). *Supporting emotional needs of the gifted.* Retrieved January 22, 2024. www.Sengifted.org

Sravanti, L. (2017). Goodness of fit. *Indian Journal of Psychiatry*, 59(4), 515.

Tortora, S. (2017). The dancing dialogue: The role of the unspoken and the creative arts in therapeutic change with infants, children, and their families. *Journal of the American Academy of Child & Adolescent Psychiatry*, 56(10), S56–S57. https://doi.org/10.1016/j.jaac.2017.07.221

Van Der Kolk, B. A. (2014). *The body keeps the score: Brain, mind, and body in the healing of trauma.* Penguin Books.

Villines, Z. (2021). What is "body doubling" for ADHD? *Medical News Today.* www.medicalnewstoday.com

Wang, X., Li, Y., Qian, Y., Cao, Y., Shriwas, P., Zhang, H., & Chen, X. (2017). Extracellular ATP, as an energy and phosphorylating molecule, induces different types of drug resistances in cancer cells through ATP internalization and intracellular ATP level increase. *Oncotarget*, 8(50), 87860.

Winnicott, D. W. (1963). Dependence in infant care, in child care, and in the psychoanalytic setting. *The International Journal of Psycho-Analysis*, 44, 339–344.

Chapter 6

Integrated/Embodied Therapy – How This All Works

Vignette 1: You May Move

"You may decide to move your arms."

– Dr. Lori Baudino to Betty, age 5

Betty stood behind her mother when starting our therapy sessions. While she appeared not to move, I witnessed her tensed hands clasped around her mother's leg, her heart beating, her eyes darting around the room, and her breath shallow. Instead of saying, "You should move," I gave permission: "You may move." I modeled stretching my arm toward Betty and her mother holding a familiar object, a clean white tissue.

Instantly, Betty peeked her head out from behind her mother's leg and looked down at her arms as they lifted toward the tissue I held out to her. She grabbed the tissue and watched it move in a swaying motion as if mesmerized by the fluidity of this soft, flowing material. This commonly used item became the transitional object that enabled Betty to communicate her feelings.

She increased her range of movement as she tossed the tissue back and forth with her mother, tearing pieces of it, and twisting it around her hands. She even hid her body under it. Her mother communicated that this was "the first time in weeks" that Betty had talked and moved out from behind her mother's legs. This was also the first time her mother saw Betty initiate her own ideas, take control, and engage curiously with another person. Betty was able to laugh and express her interest in playing and moving with her mother and with me.

With permission to move, this seemingly shy, withdrawn child was given a space to connect. Betty's developmental challenges inhibited her movement and confidence in the world, but permission and use of a transitional object to facilitate movement transformed her inability into capability.

When using movement in a therapeutic session, parents, educators, and medical professionals ask me, "What if the child *can't* move? What if they

DOI: 10.4324/9781003363491-7

feel like they can't dance?" I become the crusader of all things movement, dedicated to informing the masses that everything we do in life involves motion. From our heart beating to how we explore the world around us, movement is the dance that creates connection, communication, and growth.

Vignette 1 Intervention: You May Move

Activity Prompt: Follow the activity prompt within the clinical session: Find a familiar object such as a tissue, glove, paper, or scarf. Explore the many ways this object can move. With your permission, play and analyze the speed at which you and the provider manipulate the object, such as twisting, ripping, throwing, and swaying. Even find ways to connect holding the object together with the provider. Have the provider follow your lead by moving the way you move and then you can move the way the provider moves too.

Provider Note: *As discussed throughout the book, the simplicity of moving together with a transitional object promotes increased safety and connection. Notice if the child you are working with has an expansive range of ideas or a limited, rigid mindset. Repeat this activity throughout your treatment time to promote an increased range of ideas, flexible thinking, and increased connection. Following the child's lead, you acknowledge each movement choice while also incorporating magnifying the movement (bringing intensity and expansion) or minimizing it (making it smaller and more subtle).*

Vignette 2: Setting Intentions

"What if I mess up or I can't change how I feel? What if I am not good enough?"

– David, age 13

Each week that I met with David, he had another fixed idea of his life, interactions, and feelings. He sat stiffly with his head down, his shoulders rolled back, and shortened breath. So I focused first on his body, not his words.

We explored how to replace his rigid position with ease. "David, what do you want out of today's session?" I asked to set an intention. David communicated that he wanted more energy and more options to get through his day so he could feel relaxed and breathe again.

We started the process by using our bodies to act out his current state. We exaggerated our postures to increase this tension, tightness, and shortness of breath. This was difficult to do; naturally, our bodies wanted to relax, to breathe. But we felt appreciative that our bodies knew how to respond. Every time we tightened, there was a reciprocal loosening. We explored these opposites in our motions. David could move his body many ways, but I asked him to find a final posture that felt most comfortable for today. He chose to stand with his arms and legs outstretched like a star. He stood secure in his pose, appearing free and open. His ability to push past his comfort zone and explore his options gave him a better understanding of his intentions.

David felt energized. He had stabilized his breathing and increased awareness of his body by participating in a relational movement experience. David was also able to identify his needs and see a positive transformation in his choices and capabilities.

Vignette 2 Intervention: Setting Intentions

Activity Prompt: Explore the following prompt within the clinical session: Think about a non-preferred feeling or event. Notice where you experience this idea in your body. Explore playing with the tension and release of this area in your body. Can you realize your choices to move or change the feeling state and ultimately find resolution and comfort?

Provider Note: *Placing the challenged concept onto the body is another way to invite acceptance of feelings and a sense of control. Tension and release exercises of the muscles are helpful relaxation techniques used for emotional support. This activity promotes an intentional feeling of the body and a child's choices within their feeling states.*

Vignette 3: True Triumph

"I can't change my feelings, I have something wrong with me."

– Carlos, age 9

When a child is stuck in a pattern of disbelief and feels he cannot change his feelings, we begin the sessions by looking at how this mindset is embodied and what purpose this state serves him.

"What is this problem doing for you?" I asked Carlos. His body posture turned from tight withheld arms and a flat facial affect to a droop. Carlos folded in half and moved around the floor slowly, as if he were searching for an answer. He didn't make eye contact at this point, as he had done when he first stated his problem to me. As I watched his body, I could see that he had developed a pattern of embodying his problems (i.e., consistently stating he felt stuck, and physically creating challenging postures, movements, and affect to match this problematic state). The congruence within his body with his verbal communication appeared to validate his perspective and provide a way to control his surroundings. If he wasn't working on a problem, then he felt he might not be seen or taken care of, which would feel very chaotic and scary for him, per his report.

I first honored his preferred state by having him stay in this kneeling, "melted" position instead of changing or standing upright. I mirrored his movements with my body melting into position with my arms and shoulders rounded and pointing toward the ground. We explored together by moving in ways that felt even messier, holding onto various materials such as scarves to mix color, shape, and directions. We took turns following one another and trying out different ideas all that felt challenging in tension, posture, and dynamic (i.e., holding a balancing pose or contorting our body in challenging ways). Ultimately, Carlos found a way to independently create new ideas and change his pattern into solutions out of his postures or by physically relaxing his shoulders and lightly jumping around the therapy room. With his ability to control his movements, he followed suggestions with curiosity and excitement instead of discontent or conflict.

Carlos relayed feeling more confident in his abilities and his health. He couldn't think of a single problem at that moment. He said, "I kind of feel fixed." We laughed as if he had never been broken and smiled knowing he now had options to repair and grow from within and through his relationship to himself and others.

Vignette 3 Intervention: True Triumph

Activity Prompt: Explore the following prompt within the clinical session: Think about a current problem. Can you reenact it in your body? What happens to your shoulders? Are they moving slowly or quickly? Explore how this movement posture serves you. Can you notice if this brings you closer to another person (the therapist or parent) or gives you space to be separate? Does having this problem provide you with permission to be cared for or shut out? As the witness the provider will support the resolution by responding to whichever purpose the movement has evoked. (i.e., if you need to be cared for – the provider will hold hands, have a snack, breathe with you; If needing separateness – the provider will join you in drawing independently, or by sitting and listening to a song).

Provider Note: *In this activity, you get to respond to the purpose of the movement congruently. Modeling the requested intention for the child will help the child symbolize what is congruent to their needs and wants. Help the child notice their intentions by looking at what their body does at that moment – i.e., how they sit, where they are looking, etc., breaking down each part of their movements not by talking but by physically trying on the movement and joining them in the exploration.*

Vignette 4: Can You See the Dysregulation?

"How do I know when my child is going to flip out or disconnect?"
– Parent of Julia, age 5

Children have the ability to sustain attention and increase their focus. This is achieved when the right body posturing and movement sequence has occurred. Julia had a diagnosis of attention deficit disorder and a presentation of being twice exceptional (her intellectual achievements ranked high above her age level and presentation which created developmental and behavioral challenges).

When Julia appeared at her most calm, she was sitting upright at her table playing with toys or drawing. When she was dysregulated (not organized or comfortable in her body), she would fall to the ground or run to and from other adults and children.

In the therapeutic setting, we explored how to identify these movement planes, or dimensions, in order to support the "just right" states of engagement for her. Her parents could see that when she started to lower her body to the ground on a vertical plane (head to feet), she needed support. When she moved to and from sagittally, she also needed their support.

Next, we practiced intentionally moving in these dimensions. We started by supporting Julia to use the horizontal plane for regulation. The horizontal plane was explored by providing parallel play with toys, moving side to side, rocking, and rolling trains. Each sequence of interacting with Julia took the following order. First, we would move from side-to-side horizontally playing, then moving into a sitting-up position we transitioned to tabletop games or drawing. We would stand vertically to move to the table and complete the presented activities. Then finally we would move toward one another in passing, turn-taking, problem-solving, within the sagittal plane. I would verbalize to Julia and her parents the movement planes we were exploring and support a discussion of examples of when Julia moved in these different ways during emotional states.

Now, Julia's parents communicate that Julia's movements and reactions feel more predictable in nature (they can observe what plane she is in and what she needs to do in order to move into regulation), ultimately supporting an increase in their family communication and connection.

Vignette 4 Intervention: Can You See the Dysregulation

Activity Prompt: Follow the provided prompt and questions to continue the integrative movement practices: Explore planes of movement. Flip the order of the planes by starting in the sagittal dimension. Move forward and back and notice if this feels safe or intrusive. What is missing? Explore in the vertical dimension – become the leader and assert yourself. Close the activity by partnering to parallel play or relax in a mindfulness breathing or stretching exercise.

Provider Note: *Using the planes and passing the control to the child allows you to see the progress made throughout clinical care. Exploring the dimensions is another opportunity to bring parents and family into the session to explore together. You may also invite writing, drawing, props, and music to increase the experience and documentation.*

Vignette 5: For Laughter, Play, and Love for All

> *"Patrick loves playing the same games and hearing the same story over and over and over again."*
>
> – Father of Patrick, age 8

When Patrick would play at home, he would repeatedly ask his father to tell him the same story about his favorite beach vacation. He took out the same toys and replayed the same story repeatedly. At first, his parents thought this would pass, but they became worried he was stuck. And what did that mean?

In sessions, we explored many sequences that occurred in the play. We identified the meaning behind Patrick's need for mastery, playing out themes he had not fully learned or understood. For instance, the story he preferred had consistent organization (i.e., packing up the car for the trip). He then identified the fast pace of the car ride and the waves at the beach, activities that he felt were unpredictable and out of his control. While his parents had been concerned about his fixed mindset and repetitive play, they began to understand how each choice he made was meaningful. They learned how to expand on these themes of organization and control. All together, we used movement to embody the various actions in the story: Moving in an organized pattern or rushing and jumping in waves.

As Patrick's parents began to better understand, they joined in movements to embody the story completely. Patrick was then able to share control of the story and make changes in his play, even creating completely new ideas.

His parents now saw the value in the underlying themes explored in the story and how they could use the qualities of movement, such as speed and timing, to help Patrick have more opportunities to share his ideas and be accepted in his needs.

Vignette 5 Intervention: For Laughter, Play, and Love for All

Activity Prompt: The provider will model and explore the following activity within the clinical session or reference as an activity for the child/parent to explore at home: Think about an event that may feel challenging (or just seems to keep reappearing, a story you keep retelling over and over). Use toys, art, and, most importantly, your body to retell the events. See if you can embody the speed, the facial expressions, and the body posture. Play with the opposites. Take the same scenario and see if your body can move differently (i.e., how could a superhero respond, a baby, or grandma).

Provider Note: *Identifying a challenging and reoccurring topic can be explored verbally or noted throughout sessions. Using creative tools such as art, toys, and movement invites more learning opportunities through play and represents the session's themes. Using opposites allows for more options, expansion, and transformation for the child as he/she/they develop more coping skills and insights.*

Vignette 6: Are You Aware?

"My child can communicate, share feelings, and socialize even though she was diagnosed on the autism spectrum. But how do I ensure she is accepted?"
– Mother of Sara, age 8

Through therapeutic support, Sara's mother learned all about her daughter's strengths and adaptive responses. Sara and her mother communicated appreciation for all of Sara's passions and gifts while seeking support for her to feel accepted and understood throughout her life.

In one session, Sara came in speaking about her interest in horses and her weekend with her family. She sat across from me and moved her legs in a trotting fashion as if she were a horse. She would frequently describe her passions with her whole body, moving in patterns and expressing qualities she had observed in other animals and people.

But what was *her* preference for moving? How did she interact in her world as Sara?

During one particular session, she and I wanted to explore her preferences versus her movements mirroring her horses. We used a prop called a "body sock," an incredibly soft and stretchy spandex-type material that she described as "a safe place to feel not judged or misunderstood." She started by breathing and then followed my directions to move with various qualities.

Sara realized in this session that she felt more comfortable moving with lightness. She felt like she was graceful and would be perceived as more friendly if she wasn't forceful, which might appear like aggression. She had immediate interpretations of how people would perceive her because of her diagnosis. Her autism diagnosis and these basic ways of moving created a stereotype and potentially made others judge her.

I offered her a way to join with me to create movement with strength that wasn't aggressive but rather, assertive, and strong. She could use a full range of movements in our space together, safe, accepted, and seen as what she described as "feeling normal and free."

The use of movement provided insight into Sara's emotional experiences with others: How she felt judged, her preferences, and desire to feel accepted. Movement acts as a parallel process to real-life challenges and an outlet for resolution and acceptance.

Vignette 6 Intervention: Are You Aware?

Activity Prompt: Explore the following activity prompt within the clinical session: Take an opportunity to move with props. For example, scarves, blankets, pillows, tissue, or even a body sock. Explore different movement qualities such as speed, direction, and the quality of weight (moving with strength or light floaty movement). Notice which qualities feel the best to you or how you may be perceived moving this way.

Provider Note: *Props allow for a safe exploration separate from the body, as the material becomes a transitional object. Additionally, using effort qualities invites exploration and a rich understanding of the child's needs and preferences. Lastly, awareness develops when you support the child to notice how others perceive their body (family, yourself, the clinician).*

Vignette 7: Replace Distraction With Empowerment

"She won't stop crying . . . just give her a toy."
— Care provider for Rebecca, age 18 months

When I met Rebecca, she started to cry whenever another person held her or her family left the room. When she cried, she was immediately given distractions such as toys or entertainment provided by an adult.

I guided Rebecca's parents to watch and observe her body movements. These observation skills would enable them to anticipate Rebecca's response and give them time to communicate a plan accordingly.

Her parents observed the tension in her shoulders, fists, and face, but they noticed that she could easily shift into smiling and slow down her breath when they gave her time. The transitions became quicker and less stressful after Rebecca anticipated her family's actions and trusted them to return to her. Within our therapeutic sessions, I supported the family to see Rebecca as competent and capable. They didn't need to always resort to distraction when she exhibited a feeling. Therapy taught Rebecca's parents to notice that her reactions were merely a response to the change and not that she was in distress or harmed. They could empower her to choose how to say goodbye instead of crying. Her parents could acknowledge these changes while still honoring their transition out the door.

Therapeutic interventions using movement and the body are powerful and effective in aiding children who struggle to communicate, further fostering secure transitions and loving attachment between child and parent.

Vignette 7 Intervention: Replace Distraction With Empowerment

Activity Prompt: The following directive is provided to support empowerment and to reduce transitional challenges. Follow the provided concept and offered here: Next time you react by being upset to a new experience or a transition such as your parent leaving the room, the provider/therapist can support you by responding as if you had given a compliment. The provider or the parent will learn to gesture to you an appreciation for you sharing your feelings, and they will reflect on how they, the adult, will feel when they are gone, while also providing you with options of what you can do while they are gone. Invite your parents or the therapist to show you how this will work and have them practice with you by using a big smile, waving, and expressing the safety of the situation. For instance, you can role-play your parents' encouragement saying, "Mommy's walking to the car. You can sing, wave, and draw a picture."

Provider Note: *Empowerment is about matching the child's timing and identified need by emphasizing the adult's appreciation and experience of the change (i.e., the transition, separation, distance). Make sure the choices provided are all doable and available. Make sure to replace isolation with confirmed love and appreciation for one another-attachment is a positive relational dynamic.*

Vignette 8: Building Trust

> *"My dad won't let me do that. He says I'm too little. He says that about everything I try."*
>
> – Anaya, age 5

Anaya and her father came to sessions in hopes of understanding and enhancing their communication skills. Her father felt that she didn't listen to him when she immediately dismissed his requests. Meanwhile, Anaya felt like she was not good at anything, always feeling criticized by her dad, and not allowed to accomplish tasks independently. Her dad was always telling her what to do before she had a chance to do it on her own. Clearly, they had been misunderstanding each other.

In one session, we worked to build trust and identify how likely each one could support the other. I had them face each other with their hands touching. First, Anaya was asked to put her weight onto her father, then her father would have a turn to place his weight against her hands, and then to find a mutual way to hold each other. This sharing and turn-taking in support provided an embodied experience of their relational challenges of trust.

Anaya and her dad could not figure out how to support each other in this activity. Anaya became upset when her dad leaned on her. Her dad became upset when Anaya tried to direct him. They communicated that this was too much but remained open to trying to build trust.

Just a few weeks later, after they had begun sharing control and implementing new strategies at home, they could see how they both loved being co-leaders. Now, when we explored the same activity, Anaya was able to shift her posture and ultimately felt supported by her father. While having to physically support her father was challenging because he was much bigger than she, Anaya realized that if she were next to her dad, he could lean on her, and she could hold him without falling over. Finally, they were directed to find a mutual position to sit in, and they immediately decided to hug. They held each other with equal weight and directionality – both bodies securely held together as in an embrace, with their attention focused inward on each other.

The therapeutic session allowed for time to process the movement experience through drawing and discussion. Anaya and her father collaborated to identify their preferences for being supported and independent. The symbolism in this nonverbal exercise helped them identify their relationship patterns and change their communication for the better. The use of the body to hold and trust each other allowed them to feel their own body boundaries (independence and strength) while also connecting to the other (vulnerability and security).

Vignette 8 Intervention: Building Trust

Activity Prompt: Follow the provided activity prompt within the clinical sessions: With your family members, take turns facing each other and attempt to hold/balance one another by pressing your hands together and shifting your weight for pressure into your hands for stability. Explore what it feels like to have one person hold the other. You might see that holding hand to hand might feel unstable. Explore different ways to work (i.e., back-to-back, shoulder-to-shoulder, lying down, using the wall). Most importantly, each of you give suggestions and try them out. Finding a way that simultaneously feels like both of you have support and control. The interaction might look like a hug or a secure bridge. Write and draw about how the experience and observation relate to your family dynamic and individually.

Provider Note: *Balancing and holding postures within a family dynamic will elicit emotional experiences and patterns reminiscent of the connections. As the provider, you will observe dynamics related to control, power, sharing, and acceptance dynamics. Ensure safety by setting a specific time to explore each posture. Ensure that each partner is available and ready before taking the weight of the other person's body.*

Vignette 9: What Is Your Kryptonite?

"I feel I've lost all my power and am defeated when I am misperceived or ignored."

– Dr. Lori Baudino

Several of the children I work with have asked me to share with them my personal "kryptonite": An experience of a person, action, or item that makes me feel weak, unresponsive, and powerless. By sharing my own kryptonite, the children smile that they know me in an authentic and mutual way and more so that they are not alone in having these experiences. This is a wonderful moment to reflect on how insightful children can be and how they are able to offer opportunities to process feelings collaboratively.

In one session, a client, Chantelle identified her kryptonite as "when I feel I am mean or ugly," highlighting her own self-doubt and criticism, which makes her feel powerless. In another session with a client, Mateo stated that his kryptonite was "when a teacher yells at me with a big voice that I feel is mean." The examples continued from one child session to another, with the therapeutic setting enabling each child to realize the range of incredible feelings and body sensations that occur when we are confronted with certain events and/or relationships. In each session, the child and I collaborated to help one another find the power to be strong from within. We sought our own truths, asked one another for help, and problem-solved strategies to break apart our kryptonite so it couldn't be used against us anymore.

Children enjoy when emotional expressions and psychological topics are filled with movement, play, and relatable topics. One therapeutic strategy I often use is called "super senses," as in *our* superpowers, which provide awareness of a child's sensory system so they have options for defeating their kryptonite (insecurities/punitive experiences) and making their world feel safer.

Super senses are used to support children to identify a sensory strength to feel more comfortable in a situation. For instance, a child feeling overwhelmed by noises in a large classroom may use their superpowered eyes to look around and see their peers' facial expressions, surrounding colors, and shapes. Similarly, a child feeling uncomfortable due to excessive visual stimulation from screens, people, or lights may focus on the super sense of

---

Vignette 9 Intervention: What Is Your Kyptonite?

Activity Prompt: Follow the provided prompt within the clinical session or provide as an exploration for the child/parent to use at home: Explore your sensory superpowers. Identify the senses; sight, taste, touch, sound, etc. Identify verbally or write with family members what sensory experience seems to flood you most. Now think about an opposing super sense. For instance, the next time you become upset that your house is too loud with all your siblings and parents talking, change your auditory experience by increasing your visual experience – put on your favorite sunglasses, look outside the window, or observe your family members smiling faces.

> **Provider Note:** *Sensory superpowers are another way to empower options and a sense of control. You can model using the same sense to zoom in and out of the situation (i.e., visual overwhelm can be met by visually focusing on see-ing a child smiling, or overwhelming noise can be supported with alternative sounds). Consequently, a sense can be adjusted to an alternative (i.e., replace overwhelmed sounds with a soft preferred texture). You can write these options out with the child or family to support for times outside of therapy.*

touch to feel comforted by soft textures or smooth surfaces. The important piece to remember here is to support children in being mindful to use their senses so they can feel their best in all situations.

Vignette 10: Embodied Planning

"I'm not used to making my own decisions. I don't know where to start or how to make the right choice."
– Robert, age 15

Robert sat quietly with his head down. He made minimal eye contact and appeared uncomfortable when asked any basic question, such as his inter-ests or his age. Robert did, however, move.

When I entered the room, he smiled and looked at me. He started to move his fingers, tapping them together in a sequence. He looked like he was playing the piano or typing. I asked if I could play too. Together we moved our fingers. Robert increased the speed of tapping, changing up the sequencing and patterns. He appeared to be having a great time testing me and challenging me.

I narrated that we seemed to be making plans. I admired his ideas and his interest in moving and dancing with his fingers. He stated that he liked having a plan but wasn't used to making decisions on his own. I pointed out how his finger movements had a beginning, middle, and end – that he had been making a plan the entire time.

I gave Robert permission to decide how to move, but also asked him to follow my lead and share control. This movement activity developed into a body experience that helped him realize he was capable of making deci-sions (decisions that felt right to him), and he could take this same ability and steps for making any decision. He also learned how to explore options, ask for help, and trust himself.

Through this lighthearted intervention, I was able to empower Robert and support him in developing strategies to better assert himself and make choices. Making plans can be a stifling process, especially for someone who fears making the right choice. Movement is an innate way to communicate, and with awareness, we can spring into action.

Vignette 10 Intervention: Embodied Planning

Activity Prompt: Explore the following prompt within the clinical sessions or provide for the child/parent to use at home: When you feel overwhelmed by the to-do list of everyday expectations and parental demands. Instead of just talking through, allow the opportunity to create a movement sequence to showcase each task. Notice which movement feels best first, second, and last. Did you move the way you had planned the events to go? Listen to your body to help you clarify and organize your step-by-step plans.

Provider Note: *Exploring planning through movement allows a playful spin on those typical mundane, tedious, and sometimes overwhelming demands. Children learn through play and movement. You may model examples of what a task you do looks like and then have the child have a turn. Additionally, invite parents and other family members to join the session. Movement can include role-playing, gestures, facial affect, and creating a movement dance of each task the child completes.*

Vignette 11: Love Languages for Children

"My child pushes away when I try to hold her (hug) at the end of the day, and especially when she is upset."

– Mother of Jennifer, age 6

Six-year-old Jennifer's parents typically rushed to her aid whenever she fell. They held her and moved quickly to ensure her safety. But Jennifer had a different response to her parents: Instead of viewing their quick and direct measures as ways to feel secure, she pulled away from them. She pushed, screamed louder, and even found ways to hide when she was hurt.

Jennifer was actually receptive to being held, but the question of how to be approached was the most important piece in learning more about her needs and ways to support her. When her parents saw her reaction, they intensified their approach and tried to get to her quicker. Then, after she pulled away, they would ignore her and go about their day. Jennifer reported in therapy that she wanted hugs but that her parents running at her made her feel uncomfortable, even scared. Communication clearly needed to be reset.

During family sessions, we worked to identify each person's needs and preferences. We explored in movement various timings (how fast and slow to move toward and with one another) and the weight of their body interactions (holding gently or with firmer contact). Each family member communicated stories and memories of preferences and nonpreferred interactions. Together they worked to identify a need for slowing down before embracing, using eye contact to indicate to Jennifer that they were approaching, and to keep the body contact feeling firm and secure. Ultimately, they all communicated clearly, and Jennifer got the much needed and appropriate support she responded to.

This family's dynamic and emotional experience touched upon the theory of love languages that can be applied to children. Parents often want to know how to figure out which language truly fits their children. How can they provide the appropriate affection/response at the "correct time" for their specific child? Movement can be an incredible lens through which to explore and ultimately learn how to best approach your children.

Vignette II Intervention: Love Languages for Children

Activity Prompt: The provider will model the following activity within the clinical session: With your permission, explore different ways to connect with your family or with the provider. Explore moving quickly toward one another versus slowly walking up to one another. With safe hands, decide whether a grasp feels better light and soft versus firm and secure. Use words and facial expressions to indicate and cue you on what each person's body is about to do.

Provider Note: *Exploring love languages is based on the work of Gary Chapman (Chapman, 2010). The main intention here is to support the awareness of the many ways we feel and express love. Connection is felt in the body and viewed instantly when exploring with movement. Use visuals of connections (puzzle pieces, links, animals cuddling, etc.) to evoke more learning options.*

Vignette 12: Imagery in Motion

> *"How can I connect with my child?"*
> — Mother of Ella, age 10

In this session, I provided ten different visual cards for the child, Ella, and her mother. I had created these cards by downloading, printing, and laminating images I felt pertained to the dynamic I was exploring with this particular child and parent. Each card portrayed a different image of connection, such as a puzzle piece, two people embracing, a team huddling together, and a person resting on a pillow. Ella's mother chose the card with the image of the embrace while Ella chose the card with the puzzle piece. Then we explored how our bodies could create these images through movement.

First, we considered how the puzzle pieces would look between our hands: Could they embrace each other or link together? Next, we tried to use different parts of our bodies such as our legs, feet, hips, and head. How could these body parts link and embrace? Ella and her mother smiled and generated more ideas. Ella initiated the linking and embracing of her mother's arms, legs, and head. Her mother smiled and followed Ella's lead. This ultimately led to them hugging and smiling. Just like the puzzle pieces, they fit perfectly together.

Vignette 12 Intervention: Imagery in Motion

Activity Prompt: Explore the following activity prompt within the clinical session: Using images to create movement and connection. Find pictures online, get a book or magazine, or even play cards. Join with the provider or a family member to create movement from the image. For example, connect through expressing with the body, as seen in the pictures. Additionally, expand by sharing images of animals, water, and nature. How can you move like the pictures?

Provider Note: *This activity evokes great discussion, patterning, and information. Children can bring in images, or you can work together to find photos. Truly engage the entire body using your whole virtual or in-person room, expanding the body and increasing the range of movement with timing, weight, and speed. Notice how you can relate these movements and states of being to real-life emotional experiences. Invite parents and family members to try this activity at home.*

It was delightful to see this parent and child create opportunities for intimacy by honoring their own choices, sharing them with each other, and joining together. The ability to move together promoted this possibility. Both had the permission they needed to connect with the other.

Vignette 13: When Holding Is the Answer

"We can't hold her all the time. We need to give her tough love so she can stop crying."

– Patrick, father of Sophie, age 18 months

Patrick told me he didn't want to hold Sophie because he thought it would create dependence. I immediately acknowledged that our common goal was to support her by establishing a secure bond. This ultimately would provide her with tools for becoming independent.

I started by modeling for Patrick how to observe his daughter's needs to allow her to feel competent and for him to understand her responses. Observation created understanding on a body and sensory level of how Sophie responds and interacts in her environment. I provided Patrick with the following questions: When does she seek out an adult? What makes her cry? What is the duration, frequency, and intensity of her crying? What does this look like in her body?

At first, Patrick couldn't tell me any of these answers because he was equating crying with a problem and her wanting to be held as a sign of manipulation. He didn't know what was making her cry, only that she should stop. Fortunately, due to our shared goal, Patrick allowed me to engage with Sophie when she was crying. In our sessions, I held her and offered the security she needed, modeling the various ways to provide Sophie's body with the sensory-seeking input she needed to regulate and remain calm. Patrick was able to observe the relationship that formed in that moment. I altered my holding of her body (adjusting my position and responses), which were dependent on her reactions and the situational needs. Patrick began to learn the wide range of movement interactions he could share with his daughter. He realized the great benefit of observing and engaging with Sophie through movement and words.

I modeled how my interest in Sophie's needs and her trust in my predictable responses enabled her to interact more independently and significantly reduce her crying. She even started to follow my use of sign language (gestures) and short phrases to get her needs met.

The fear of being manipulated or increasing unwanted behavior such as incessant crying can certainly cause enough distress for a parent or caretaker to want to run far away from the "needy" child. But when we give a moment for observation, movement, posture, and holding, a connection is formed and a space is provided for security, soothing, and independence.

Vignette 13 Intervention: **When Holding Is the Answer**

Activity Prompt: Use the following prompt to create connection and insight for clinical care: As the parent, take a quiet moment to observe your child's movements. See if you can write down the observed movement qualities with paper and a pen. When the child is calm and relaxing or sharing a significant response, can you notice what part of their body they use? Explore these questions: Is this movement fast or slow? Does the movement last a long time? Are there any repetitive movements (for instance, clapping arms, kicking legs, and rubbing eyes)? Do you know what this movement means? Does the child always move this way? Observing a child gives you a view into their predictable patterns and how they interact in the world.

Provider Note: *You can reassess a child's movement patterns throughout your treatment planning and sessions. Invite parents to explore watching and observing at home and in your sessions. Explore by providing a written form for the parent to fill out during your sessions as they watch and wonder about their child's meaningful movements and emotional themes.*

Vignette 14: Is Body Movement Communication?

"Talk to the doctor – look at her when she is talking."

– Father of Daisy, age 4

When entering a doctor's office, a place of work, or in the company of an adult, we often feel obligated to ensure that our children show respect. This respect is defined for our children as sitting still, responding to any and all questions, and making eye contact.

For me, this is not imperative. I encourage parents to understand that the therapeutic environment is a unique place that allows their child to be exactly as they are, a place where I can communicate and listen to them with their gestures, posture, facial expressions, and nonverbal communication.

When four-year-old Daisy entered my office, she walked backward with her body facing her father. She made no eye contact and said nothing. She walked with care and coordination, managing to balance her limbs without bumping into the desk or door. She gently lowered her body onto the shag carpet and faced the couch, continuing to look at her father's face.

I said,

> Welcome, Daisy and Dad. I am going to tell you about our time together today. Daisy, I was able to watch you carefully walk into the room facing your dad. I see how you are sitting on the floor, how you are making choices in touching the pillows and playfully moving the fabric.

I informed Daisy and her father that it was Daisy's choice to talk. She could decide to use words, look in the direction that felt best for her, and that her father could talk with me too. After her father answered and asked some preliminary questions, I noticed Daisy's speed of movement increased. She flipped pillows upside down and backward.

In the way dance/movement therapists practice, I joined Daisy. I asked her father to see if he could observe his daughter's movements and view them as intentional, so we could speak her language rather than assuming she was being disrespectful (facing backward, not looking at my face or answering with words, at the start) to me, the "doctor."

We turned the pillows, moved our arms, and followed her ideas and nonverbal language. I gave permission to Daisy to take turns being the leader, but she decided at first to stay the leader and have control. Ultimately, by giving her this secure opportunity, she was then able to shift to follow her father, intentionally turned around, watched, and followed me.

Together we created a routine and a conversation of how our power dynamic would occur in this session. Daisy would be in charge since she had a lot to offer. She used space to bond with her father and opened up when she felt ready.

To me, this ten-minute moment opened the stage for an authentic relationship, highlighted the dynamics that Daisy creates in social situations, and offered insight into her processing and connections. The trust was immediately created, and the therapeutic alliance secured.

Vignette 14 Intervention: Is Body Movement Communication?

Activity Prompt: Explore the following prompt within the clinical sessions: Be joined with non-verbal language. When entering a new situation or simply practicing your movement language, start by following your rhythm, how fast or slow you are moving, and see if you can be joined by the provider or a family member as you move your arms and fingers and which way your body is facing. Pretend you are entering different social situations. How might you pretend to walk in a large group of people, visit a doctor's office, or visit a relative? Explore different ways to sit, smile, nod, or use words.

Provider Note: *Posturing and facial affect are key to social communication and connection. Supporting a practice space for emotional expression and recognizing various etiquette and situational dynamics fosters opportunities for successful relationships and safety in the child's interactions. You can ask the child for examples from their real life or model scenarios you know the child may experience during their development. Not only can we instruct our children on social etiquette, but we can also practice our body movements.*

Vignette 15: Soothing the Busy Day

> *"How do you get your children to nap and go to sleep on time?"*
>
> – Mother of two, ages 2 and 6

Parents often ask me how to get their children to nap and rest. I believe we can learn about sleep and what soothes your child in the early months and then watch as changes occur during development. Let me explain.

Six-year-old Robbie and two-year-old Victoria had a busy daily routine, including time at home, school, sports, play, eating, and homework. The question of where to fit in time to nap was tricky. First, I needed to learn about their preferences. While observing their playtime together, I noticed that physical touch soothed Victoria, and Robbie seemed most calm when he was listening to directives or music. I started by helping them develop a plan that each could use to relax.

I encouraged their mother to allow Victoria time in a space filled with comfy blankets and tactile objects she could enjoy touching (she even tried giving Victoria a massage). While, Robbie was given an auditory listening activity. Their mother massaged Victoria's back while asking the children to focus on their head, nose, ears, shoulders, etc. Listing the parts of the body and what and where to focus soothed both children. At first, the naps were only three minutes long, but quickly, the children started asking for

---

Vignette 15 Intervention: Soothing the Busy Day

Activity Prompt: Follow the activity prompt within your clinical sessions or provide the activity to the parent/child to utilize at home: Explore your soothing preferences. Get support for both your parents and you by identifying how you find relief and recovery. Explore if relaxing comes from listening to a book, song, or yoga nidra. Or do you seem to play with your hair or blankie or want to be held? Having your parents and you know your preferences for soothing is the key to helping you fall asleep or rest.

> **Provider Note:** *Explore with the parents' ways in which they can observe their child's soothing, calm states. Explore their birth story and early years to assist in knowing the child's preferences and patterns. Identify the sensory component of soothing, sights, textures, smells, and sounds. Ultimately, start with the preferred way of soothing the child. Then introduce alternative options by pairing a new soothing/coping intervention with the original. For instance, if the child calms by listening to music, then pair music with a transitional object (stuffed animal) and then fade the music out or vice versa. Increasing a child's tool kit for soothing supports daily living, transitions, and life changes. Supporting a parent to know their child's regulatory needs will help the child successfully sleep and relax. Some children need stimulation, input, or even revved-up experiences to regulate before falling asleep. In contrast, others need soothing, slower, and more calming spaces with minimal distractions. All options are welcome and celebrated, as this is the child's beginning adaptive skill for survival!*

more time. Soon the entire family was taking thirty to forty-five minute breaks to regroup and rejuvenate.

We expanded on how to wind down on the go, such as in the car, waiting in line, or at a busy dinner. Having a moment to check in with their senses and be aware and present in their body allowed them all to feel calm and connected to one another. Their mother communicated a new appreciation for long, busy days, knowing she and her children could have more moments to recover with ease.

Vignette 16: Teenage Transformation

"I can't get any space. Everyone is always around."

– Bonnie, age 16

Bonnie was always surrounded by care providers, siblings, and other family members while undergoing treatment at the hospital. She acknowledged that, while she felt loved, she had a hard time asking for her own space. I suggested that we play a movement activity with her brother and dad. She stood with her arms on her hips and her feet together. I asked her dad to fill in the "negative space," or any of the surrounding space beside Bonnie's pose. Bonnie's dad walked over and stood close to his daughter with his hand through the side of her arm.

He was asked to freeze and wait as Bonnie moved aside, watching her dad standing in the middle. Her brother then entered the space and stood an arm's distance away with his hands in the air.

They each took turns filling in the space surrounding the various poses they created. Bonnie soon realized that the smaller she made her stance, the closer her family came together. The more clear she was in her posture, the more distance she was granted.

This movement exploration allowed family members to share and communicate their needs for connection and space. They were able to practice reading each other's body cues, facial expressions, and ultimately, words to get their most desired needs met. We sat down and discussed these patterns and reviewed best practices for communicating our love while still respecting another person's space.

By taking an embodied approach and bringing knowledge to the body, the family members were able to hear one another's needs. They also could feel them, experience them, and work to incorporate a better outcome on a daily basis.

Vignette 16 Intervention: Teenage Transformation

Activity Prompt: Explore the following activity within the clinical session: Taking turns with family members, one person poses in the middle of the group. Notice any of the negative space (the space surrounding the body). For instance, between fingers, underarms, and around the head. Take turns placing each person's body into those "free spaces," creating a new pose. While holding this new position, the original posed person steps out to observe this new pose and re-enter the negative space again. Notice what postures create proximity and which allow for more distance between each person.

Provider Note: *Ask the questions: Do you notice a preference? Does your posture represent the connection or space you are desiring? You will find similarities between the visual dynamics that arise in this activity. Parents and children will get intimately close or remain separate; power dynamics will appear, and playfulness will ensue. Ensure safety by asking participants for permission before entering each other's body space. Additionally, ensure that the bodies remain not touching to increase security.*

Vignette 17: Changing the Impossible

"He doesn't move or communicate with others."

– Father of Andres, age 10

Children with severe pathology or medical complications often have psychological symptoms that manifest in the body. I observed Andres, like so many others, sitting in the outpatient clinic with a stiff posture awaiting his oncology checkup. Andres received dance movement therapy within the hospital to support his diagnosis of cancer and treatment compliance. He used gestural movements and vaguely muttered words or simple phrases to signal his needs.

I spoke to Andres just as I would to any other child, but I used a bit more humor and banter. Andres tended to roll his eyes or look away with a grin on his face. I believed he communicated a lot through his posture, his choices in gestures, and his distinct facial expressions.

I mirrored Andres's posture and movements and told him how his posture and method of breathing felt to me. I shared how his body and mind were making choices that indicated to me his memories of being in the hospital, interacting with other people, and even memories from his experiences outside the hospital. On occasions where his siblings or parents were present, I encouraged him to try moving with his family members to see what choices they each made and what memories they had to share. We would join and match his father's posture, then his sister's, and finally, my own as the therapist. We used small movements at first and then expanded from using half of our bodies to reaching and twisting motions. Andres likened his movements to an "airplane ride," a memory of a trip he had forgotten about and now was excited to revisit with his family.

He increased his range of movement and language as he described in short phrases what he recalled. His facial expressions changed, and he laughed while he synchronized his memory with his movements.

I thanked Andres for taking me on his family trip and showing me his memory. I communicated back to him all of the movements, words, and ideas I saw him express. Andres was actually a great communicator, and

---

Vignette 17 Intervention: Changing the Impossible

Activity Prompt: Explore the following activity prompt and movement interactions to support the clinical session: Starting with the simplest movements (i.e., fingers moving), make subtle shifts and then drastic changes. Notice any tightness in your lower back or throughout your body. Gradually shift your weight into that spot, allowing for control in the areas that aren't comfortable by softening them and shifting your weight. Repositioning the shoulders, knees, and feet on the ground can allow you to gain more support. While noticing, your breathing will begin to guide you in lengthening and curving your spine. This movement enables the breath to flow from the bottom of your feet to the top of your head.

> **Provider Note:** *Subtle shifting and re-posturing is a beautiful activity to invite ease and fluidity into the body. Imagine a slow-moving river or a slithering snake as the movement shifts throughout the body. Providing permission to let go of tension will increase the child's awareness and sense of control.*

through movement and connection, language emerged more comfortably, and connection was possible. By allowing Andres to see his choices through the use of motion, he was further able to access these memories and share them with his family and me.

Vignette 18: Listening With Observation

> *"How can I help my kid listen to me?"*
>
> – Patrick, father of child, age 3

Patrick communicated how frustrated he was about his son's lack of respect. He expressed that his son never looked at him when he talked, didn't listen the first time he was asked, and seemed to always have his own ideas. "How can I get him to listen?" he asked.

Utilizing dance/movement therapy techniques of mindful motion, Patrick and his son took turns moving their bodies while describing their motions to each other. They both developed a new vocabulary for identifying speed, weight, and direction (how their bodies were moving). Each became an expert observer as they asked questions and played with facial affect. They tried to decide if each could identify what the other was doing nonverbally without giving away the answer (saying the idea out loud). This playful movement became the start of truly understanding, watching, and accepting each other.

Patrick was encouraged to use this language before making a demand of his son. "I see you . . .," and "Now, let's . . . " To his amazement, Patrick communicated in our next session that his son was "listening" to him; his son actually looked at him when he asked and followed requests.

Vignette 18 Intervention: Listening With Observation

Activity Prompt: Follow this "charades 2.0" activity to support the clinical session: Taking turns, exploring using facial expressions, body postures, and gross motor movements to explore how you are feeling. Use fun, familiar themes such as a book, a movie, a sports game, or even describe a family memory. By only using the body and movement, see if you can communicate clear ideas without using words.

> **Provider Note:** *This activity is a great icebreaker game. You can also intersperse this activity within your treatment sessions to invite the opportunity to recognize the adaptations and progress made within the child's ability to communicate.*

Combining movement and communication promoted a positive connection between Patrick and his son. Patrick was able to acknowledge his son's needs and, in return, his son was able to honor his requests.

Vignette 19: Keep Playing

> *"No, I don't want to play."*
>
> – Aiko, age 5

Aiko held onto her doll without looking up. Her parents explained that she was defiant and moody, not interested in playing or communicating, even with her siblings at home since recovering from surgery and expressing increased physical pain. They felt her demeanor was alarming, and she seemed to make everyone uncomfortable.

I felt I could make a connection to Aiko's mood through her doll. Her doll became a transitional object that she held onto as if it was her security blanket. This doll, with its smiling face and sparkly dress, brought meaning to the possibility that Aiko desired to feel happy. Different from how Aiko held herself, the doll's head was propped up and smiling on her lap. Out loud I narrated, "Your head is looking down and you're sitting very still while your doll is looking up." Aiko glanced at her doll. "You two are opposites," I added. Then the movement exchange began. I told Aiko, "We will continue to move opposite from your doll. When you are ready, maybe you'll both move in the same manner too."

The opposite approach continued in movement, speed, and mood. Aiko frowned while her doll remained smiling. Aiko responded to each of my narrations with movement. She was deliberate and communicative. In other words, she had begun to play! Even as her rhythm quickened, her doll remained motionless, facing her. Finally, Aiko reached out and handed me the doll. She asked me to move with her. I took the doll and followed Aiko's movements.

By giving Aiko space and allowing her to express her resistance, she was able to understand her emotional needs through movement. We placed words to describe faces we made and increased our range of movement to share how we felt. The interaction helped Aiko develop compassion for herself. She was empowered to present the expressions and movements she wanted to without me, the therapist, telling her to act differently. Now, she had tools to experience feeling accepted in her worst mood and how to shift her feelings at her own pace.

Developing compassion, trust, and acceptance of one's feelings are key to establishing a loving connection. Whether with a transitional object or through the use of movement, a child is always communicating their inner needs and emotional desires.

Vignette 19 Intervention: **Keep Playing**

Activity Prompt: Follow the provided activity to support communication: Try using an inanimate object, a toy, (or even just your hand) to help as a transitional object. Putting the emotions, ideas, and words through this object or body part can create more ease in the exchange or interaction. This activity will allow you not to feel judged, and together you create a new world of being understood and connected. Explore if the toy car can help you brush your teeth or if a doll helps you smile when feeling sad.

Provider Note: *Using the body invites opportunities for more accessibility – supporting a transition at that moment without needing an external object. Placing the intent, blame, or response onto the object or body part removes the emotional stress on the child. It creates that easy transitional relationship and safety for trying new things or handling upsets/challenges.*

Reference

Chapman, G. D. (2010). *The five love languages.* Walker Large Print.

Chapter 7

Therapeutic Lens Explored – Perspective of Dance/ Movement Therapy

"It's weird, you know, the way so many people accept the notion that stone is inanimate, that rock doesn't move. I mean, really, this here cliff moves me every time that I see it."

(Abram, 2011)

By now, you are versed in the experience of dance/movement therapy with children – a field that has been in practice for more than fifty years – and the myriad benefits offered by this treatment model. I hope you've already adopted ways to use this lens through your clinical work and home experiences with children. As identified in "You May Move" (Chapter 6, Vignette 1), giving permission to move starts with validating the importance of movement and the body. As a practice that has been used for centuries, across cultures and diverse societies, dance and movement bring healing, connection, and communication to all. This innate way of experiencing life goes hand in hand with healing and understanding. The movement of dance is a fundamental part of human history, accompanied by ancient rituals, spiritual gatherings, and social events, and has become an integral practice for self-expression and connection throughout our world (Weber, 2022). Movement takes center stage with the Dalai Lama's dance for peace, Ellen DeGeneres's dance for cancer research and funding, and Michelle Obama's dance to aid in the fight against obesity. Dance can be the simplest sigh or large, even grandiose gestures of celebration or mourning. Its expression is whole: mind, body, and spirit.

Integration

In "Setting Intentions" (Chapter 6, Vignette 2), when a child is given permission to move, doors and windows open to options of control, release, and acceptance (Lopez, Falconer, & Mast, 2013). The premise of dance/ movement therapy is that the more expansive the movement repertoire, the more the individual becomes integrated. When we bring attention

DOI: 10.4324/9781003363491-8

to the body, we can further support the integral nature of movement and understand its scale for the child/client (see Figure 7.1). Looking at the body rather than focusing on the pathology or disease can help the child to increase their range of movement, bring flexibility and broader expression into their lives, and promote healthy exchanges. When observing a client/child, movement qualities can serve as the barometer to identify where the client/child sits on the line from chaos to rigidity. When we look at the body, we can see that the child is communicating with us (adults, caregivers) his/her/their potentially unmet needs, another expression of an adaptive response inherent to survival (Delahooke, 2019). When you use this line of measurement, the middle point is the balanced state of integration, differentiated parts that link together for function and wellness (Siegel & Bryson, 2019). I have gathered questions from hundreds of families, each referring to concern for their child's emotional regulation: The ability to remain calm and alert within their body and amid their environments.

Furthermore, the *overall* area of need for working with children falls within those two sides of the scale: chaos (a child's tantrums and disorganization) and rigidity (a child's defiance, willfulness, difficulties with change

The scale: In order for regulation to occur, integration is the key

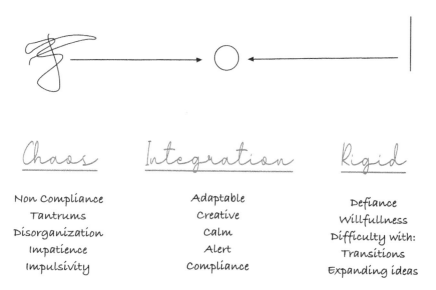

Chaos	Integration	Rigid
Non Compliance	Adaptable	Defiance
Tantrums	Creative	Willfullness
Disorganization	Calm	Difficulty with:
Impatience	Alert	Transitions
Impulsivity	Compliance	Expanding ideas

Figure 7.1 The Integration Scale

and transitions, expanding interests and ideas). All these behaviors are held in the child's body and expressed through movement – and are labeled by professionals when identifying childhood psychological and behavioral challenges. As providers, we can support integration, that ability to balance and organize sensations within the child's body, between their body and those of others (relationships), and in the wider world around them.

When children are adaptable, playful, creative, calm, and alert (focused), this is what integration looks like. An open, adaptive mindset appears to stretch for new ideas, swirl in connection to others, and grasp the larger meaning of learning and relationships. When we assess a child's words, identifying behaviors, and their movement presentation, we find more meaning behind a child's felt sense and internal state. Their posture, height, gate, and facial affect in a state of integration will be congruent rather than in opposition to their presented words. Integration is the goal for wellness to be experienced and embodied within therapeutic sessions.

The very concept of intellectual ability and adaptation lands within the body, movement and flow. Additionally, as we move our bodies, we impact and exist in relation to others. When we move with ease, we encourage others to move freely.

In quantum physics, scientists explore these themes in entanglement and the emergent property of two particles, even that of dancers in a duet impacting one another synchronistically and at a distance once they have been connected. This correlation with the science of physics continues to permeate our field of psychology, and the exploration of this impact is needed to make a change in mental health. Whether up close or at a distance, our bodies connect in physical movement, energetic vibrance, and emotional co-regulation to influence and connect (Schwartz, Stapp, & Beauregard, 2005; Vidick, 2023).

Embodied Attunement

As you integrate the lens of dance/movement therapy into therapeutic support for children, you will experience the range of movements that arise in the empathic interactions between parent and child, provider and child, and the world beyond. Again, whether it's the simple movement of breathing, a heartbeat and eye flicker, or more like jumping and twirling, all movement is both participatory and to be witnessed. In "True Triumph" (Chapter 6, Vignette 3), the child's movement choices show how he feels and senses the world while embracing the therapeutic relationship. How the body is perceived in motion and has the ability for physical expression further creates healing opportunities. By constantly linking each movement, whether big or small, in relation to how the child/client is feeling, learning occurs. In a session with a child, I can start by looking at individual movements of our fingers and quickly link them together for a sequence of movements in which a theme develops. The child plays out ideas and has a parallel process for what he/she/they is experiencing in life. Ultimately, the child gets to embody this and make choices to gain control, learn coping strategies, and have a new lived experience of connection.

Upon sharing the moving moment vignettes in this book with renowned neuroscientist Dr. Adele Diamond, the doctor smiled and stated that what she discerned in my work sounded like reciprocity or attunement – that possibly I was aligned with my clients and understood that as an important ingredient in the therapeutic relationship (Diamond, 2013). I remember retelling, "Can You See the Dysregulation?" (Chapter 6, Vignette 4), explaining that while providers fundamentally understand the importance of aligning with a child and being seen as a partner, joining in meaningful learning and connection can foster a strong therapeutic alliance. I also explained that taking the concept out of the mind (brain) and into the body (with an embodied mind) secured this connection in every therapeutic relationship I offered. (Siegel & Drullis, 2023). The embodiment of reciprocity and attunement has consistently been present within the dance/movement therapy therapeutic methodology and within my practice (Jeraka, Vidriha, & Žvelcb, 2018).

This is when being empathic doesn't just mean saying, "I see that you are sad," but rather my body is attuned to your needs. I can also move slowly if that suits the child, use weight in my steps, and direct my attention to a transitional object or topic of choice. In chemistry, "dynamic equilibrium" refers to a forward reaction that is equal to the reaction rate of the backward reaction, but the concentrations do not have to be equal (Novita, Suyono, & Yuanita, 2021). The dynamic equilibrium theory explains how reciprocity and connection create attuned partnerships. The nonjudgmental reflection of the movement presented in a session, the acceptance of the movement choices, and the direction of attention create more options and build the foundation for ongoing safe exchange. For providers, the quality of the relationship with the child/client has been linked to positive outcomes in meta-analysis across various psychotherapeutic treatments, regardless of treatment type, outcome measure, or other moderator variables (Martin, Garske, & Davis, 2000). Rightfully, a therapeutic partnership with joint learning and mutual reciprocity is indicative of high value and participation (Sandhu, Arcidiacono, Aguglia, & Priebe, 2015).

Dance/Movement Therapy for All

This book presents a valuable opportunity to explore specific aspects of child development, but I advocate for the inclusion of dance/movement therapy practices when working with any population. The research and practices of dance/movement therapy are extensive enough to assure that dance/movement therapy is suitable for any age. It may be used in business, sports, academics, as well as medical systems and across psychological needs (ADTA, 2020). In Chapter 5, the concept of the true temperature check was introduced. When we as adults understand a child's baseline and movement profile, we are granted immediate feedback on that child's psychological, social, physical, and cognitive states. In "Are You Aware?" (Chapter 6, Vignette 6), I supported the child to identify her movement patterns allowing for an accurate telling of when there was a dynamic shift that may lead to serious behaviors, actions, or psychological disruption, also known as dysregulation.

While writing this book, our world underwent a mental health crisis, so declared in 2021 by the American Academy of Child and Adolescent Psychiatry, the American Academy of Pediatrics, and the Children's Hospital Association (AACAP, 2024). Research indicates suicide is the second-leading cause of death noted by the Center for Disease Control and Prevention in ages ten to twenty-four, and those numbers have been lowered to even just five years of age (CDC, 2023). The number of children who experience mental illness, anxiety, depression, and behavioral challenges rises by the day. While the numbers are clear and have been registered across the globe, as a provider, I know this isn't unique to children today. We as a society, have long ignored, laughed at, and pushed away mental health as a field and as an imperative service for all individuals, thus unmet psychological needs are rearing up. In supporting the mental health of our children, embodied practices can be incorporated into daily care in all academic, medical, and social contexts.

I want us to think about how to find ease in our lives amid dis*ease*. In my work with children, I see how they can experience difficulty breathing, sleeping, eating, sitting still, and the list goes on. As providers and caretakers, we can offer the dance/movement therapy lens as a way to embody ease and to offer permission to move.

At pediatric hospitals, as you read in "Changing the Impossible" (Chapter 6, Vignette 17), when a patient has a *path*ology, I support a path toward viewing their responses as adaptive, in relation to their primitive instinct to assure self-preservation. To address the challenges a child or parent faces, we have the word *lens* in the word challenges for looking into how the body, mind, and spirit are interconnected and understanding that the whole child must be supported for the best results. All diseases, pathology, and obstacles in life are experienced through the body with/in movement. The moving moments collected and shared in this book are a continuation of a crusade to identify the need for pediatric, body-based mental health providers to serve as a throughline across disciplines of government, education, psychological health, and especially medical care.

As discussed in an article in the *Journal of Child Psychotherapy*,

> The door that closes on the therapy room leaves a parent behind, but at the same time allows the child's inner world to reveal itself more fully.

> There are a multitude of roles taken on by the therapist in the passage between the child's intra-psychic reality and the reality of his or her relationships with the environment.
>
> (Gvion & Bar, 2014, p. 70)

The therapeutic dynamic creates a transference between the provider, parents, and child, which can manifest as supportive, or oppositional. Furthermore, the therapeutic space between child and provider allows for an "intraConnected" (Siegel, 2022, p. 1) collaboration for revealing internal processes and embodied learning, thus producing a way to recognize chaos and rigidity and move into integration. As noted previously, the door of my therapeutic office remains open to parents, siblings, and care providers, thus establishing a micro vortex for a more macro all-encompassing collaboration. As a provider, I consider myself a conduit, a partner, and a teammate for the family, not the holder of secrets or a separate entity.

The Transitional Object

A transitional object in attachment theory identifies a mechanism the individual can manipulate, adore, and partner with to create and experience learning, relationships, and connection (Healthy Children, 2023). In the dance/movement therapy session, the transitional object becomes that of the external movement and even the space around the body as it is used in relation to another. The child experiences the opportunity to assert control in a secure and seen space, to witness self versus other, and to have safety within his/her/their experiences. Additional objects, such as scarves, toys, music, instruments, and other props (perhaps benign items found in a hospital, such as tissues) invite the child to experience new connections to the unknown and accept what is occurring in the environment of others/objects/spaces.

In dance/movement therapy, the therapist is encouraged to be at the child's level and to share ways to amplify or minimize being witness to the experience, or provide actual alternatives to the experience, depending on what is needed. I like to think of this as an ocean wave and the child's overall emotional state as an ocean (as represented in Figure 7.2). During times of heightened emotions, the provider/parent may be represented as a whale in the ocean, matching the intensity, volume, and amplification of the child's state, thus bringing attention beyond the child, as well as embracing the wave instead of overtaking it, riding with the wave through even inclement weather. Conversely, a provider/parent might represent as a small shell in the ocean, not to minimize or reject the child's state as may occur in ignoring a child's emotional state but rather bring precision, intimacy, delicacy, and consideration. The child sees this smaller modeling of their state (the parent/provider whispering, moving slower, or holding still) as a treasured shell to explore and reflect on.

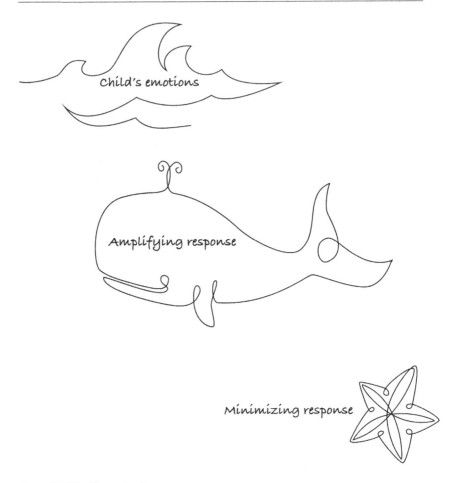

Child's emotions

Amplifying response

Minimizing response

Figure 7.2 The Ocean Analogy

Identifying Beyond Labels

Throughout this book, I've encouraged you, the provider or parent, to expand on diagnostic and social labels (i.e., lazy or aggressive) and lean toward observing children as moving, feeling, sensory beings (for example replacing lazy with observed slowness and aggression with observed dysregulation). Again, as I understand it, the concept of a diagnosis was originally intended to simplify clinical communication between practitioners and to facilitate the fluid and coherent delivery of information. Instead of speaking about a patient/client in terms of their symptoms, such as sweaty palms, racing heartbeat, perseverative speech, for instance, the provider would simply say the patient/client has anxiety. By placing the individual within the context of a single word, communication was more quickly expressed and disseminated across clinical care facilities, enabling further steps in treatment protocols. However, through this simplification, the felt experience of the word "anxiety" may get lost. Now we can broaden our communication to incorporate sensory and movement profiles and the awareness for observing the whole child: mind, body, and spirit.

We can look at the body and acknowledge that children are sensory beings: When a child feels sweaty palms or a rapid heartbeat, they can learn to understand and feel acceptance that these manifestations are true and real. When we acknowledge the body, this allows for presence and insight into the adaptive nature of felt sense, further awareness of capacities for resilience, and, finally, a transformation into what the child needs.

We exist as a higher species with feeling and movement being essential parts of who we are. As such, we can know through experience, time and time again, that feelings change and shift, that we are not defined as being mentally ill. We need to trust the innate qualities of being alive. To better trust ourselves and our felt senses, we seek information from the outside world. The collective nature of feelings, intellect, and experience leads us to sensorily interpret the world from a space that is not always apparent to our cognitive minds. There is a natural inclination to join with one another as relational beings. In a mental health crisis, there has been the shared knowledge that we are all experiencing hardship, pain, and suffering, and in that, we have all found a way to connect.

What if we choose to connect to the feeling states in our bodies? It's possible that when we feel the states of disease, pathology, and challenges, we sense a more global and collective state from our epigenetics, our birthright, and the dynamics of daily living. When we acknowledge the congruence-seeking manner in which we exist, we create an opportunity to live and embrace the child's development and our own (provider/parent) emotional needs. Embodied practices, such as dance/movement therapy, invite making a clear distinction between differentiated states of being, such as knowing the difference between our individual feelings and mental health and the broader consciousness of our society and larger world. Dance/movement therapy provides a vast range of tools and interventions to support this exploration and authentic path toward self-awareness and compassion.

A New Lens

In Chapter Two, I wrote about the use of movement planes, dimensional ways in which a child moves through the world, and how these planes represent and cue us – the provider/parents – to better understand our child's state-dependent needs and responses (Loman & Sossin, 2016). To take this further, I use the planes of movement – horizontal, vertical, and sagittal – to support parents in knowing the specific response needed to ease a child's nonpreferred response. As we work through the planes of movement, we aim to see a natural progression from one level to the next, each intended to build upon the other and increase the properties of developmental learning, meaningful connections, and integrative health. In typical development, the child's soothing connections and regulation of the horizontal plane allow for development into the vertical dimension of growth, ego strength, and skill sets. This further propels the child into the sagittal space of moving toward and away from safety and threat. The castle analogy (Chapter 4, Vignette 5), serves well to explain the dimensions of the planes, in which the horizontal represents an expansive foundation that allows for overall stability; the vertical walls are then built to allow for status, strength, visibility, and protection; finally, the drawbridge opens sagittally, allowing only the finest suitors to come in and out, thus creating opportunities for communication between safe relations and movement through the world.

In treatment, when a child barrels through the room, takes over and talks over others, I see this as moving within the sagittal plane. However, prior to these moments, the child has not moved through the prior plane dimensions and is therefore spiraling dysfunctionally and maladaptively relative to their environment; however, this behavior is also adaptive to his/her/their survival-modulational preference. Still, the child is not thriving. We can offer a vertical dimensional shift to the child by being the so-called wheel blocks or the doorframe by which to contain the rotational dimension. Being in the vertical plane supports the child to have a sense of boundaries and control established for safety. Becoming the protective provider/parental guard within the drawbridge space represents extra safety measures for securing the castle (the child). Finally, helping the child transition back to the primary horizontal plane of holding (either physical embrace or energetically) supports the child in co-regulation.

Consequently, a child asserting dominance in the vertical plane may need to be supported to move into the sagittal plane of sharing and co-leading/turn-taking or be brought back to the soothing horizontal plane for reconnection and ease, facilitating a release of the need to be in control. If the child is asserting excessive control in the vertical plane through disorganization, this may look like "bossy," "rude," or "antagonistic" behavior, but the provider/adult can still provide guidance toward the horizontal plane, supporting the child to root downward into the body or the physical room and encourage back-and-forth parallel play and exchange. This can look like joining a team to help control the space, as in "Let's look for the car keys together," or sitting on a couch and moving in a rocking manner from side to side. The planes of movement become an access point to build upward through the dimensions – horizontal, then vertical, and finally sagittal – or to realign the child by supporting recovery by returning to an earlier plane.

What I find particularly helpful is that rather than sifting through words to identify the child's presented challenge or the "correct" parental phrasing, the planes, and the map of the castle, clearly present what is accessible within our bodies. This method invites us all to observe the communication and relational paradigm as it exists rather than bringing in assumptions, labels, or overzealous interpretations. Consider each opportunity in relation to royalty, reverence, and grace. Extend the castle analogy to include the child/client as royal offspring. Build your foundation for that child by expanding outward horizontally to broaden parameters and stretch limits of learning. Build vertically from the ground into the atmosphere, manifesting a space of confidence, acceptance, and ownership and the ability to see far and wide. Finally, build a drawbridge that will open and close for only the finest suitors to enter their lives, suitors that evoke compassion, creativity, acceptance, and pure joy. And imagine that beautiful concept of treating all children with the respect of honoring their developing relationships.

Additionally, when we accept ritualistic behaviors, such as asserting control and reactivity as a coping strategy as adaptive responses to survive, we are open to the process of identifying need, supporting the environment, and accepting the whole child. For example, a child in a state of depression turns inward, away from the outside world, not to be difficult but to self-protect against adversity. When a child uses "aggressive" physicality as a defense, they should be shown how to protect via comfort, care, and connection. The action is still accepted as a means of survival, but with a new focus on safety versus harm. When we look at response/reaction as an identifier of need, we can then acknowledge that we are that higher-functioning species, equipped to handle all that comes our way.

The Brain-Body Connection

If you are like me, maybe you've come to the field of psychology motivated by a desire to help others and with a fascination with emotions and how our bodies express feelings through movement. You may have been thinking, too, "I'm not a scientist, quantum physicist, or medical doctor." Regardless, every day there are opportunities for all of us to support a child through embodied practices; we *are* actually supporting the child's brain biology (prefrontal cortex, limbic system, cerebellum, hippocampus, etc.) and scientifically promoting health.

Countless articles and books shed light on advances that occur from our brain-biology perspective (Lambert, Eisch, Galea, et al., 2019; Leisman, Moustafa, & Shafir, 2016). The same part of the brain that processes movement is the same location of learning optimization. The movement supports executive functioning skills needed for problem-solving and attention. Movement interventions support the child's individual profile (i.e., qualities of movement); regulate emotions; and increase capacities for communication, memory retrieval, and consolidation. When we move, our brain and body release necessary chemicals for supporting a positive mood, increased motivation, heightened stimulation, coping mechanisms, stress reduction, and overall morale, just to name a few. Additionally, our brains form synaptic connections for managing daily life (here/now) and enduring health that is integrated on a neurological level. Within the learning and social realms, the complex movements by which a child navigates allow for advanced thinking, reciprocity, and integration (Diamond, 2013, pp. 135–168). We know that play is an integral part of learning in early development as play encourages language development and communication skills, shared social learning, motor development, and problem-solving mastery through movement.

Childhood through adolescence is a critical time for brain development (particularly the prefrontal cortex (Arain, Haque, Johal, et al., 2013). This period brings importance to social and family interactions, which are experienced through communication, verbally and nonverbally (movement). As we can see, children live fully in their bodies. The brain's frontal lobe is responsible for decoding and comprehending social interactions. It is in this part of the mind that we empathize with others, take in nonverbal cues, learn how to read facial expressions and tones of voice, and identify the depth of human relating. Children thrive with consistent and quality time to explore concepts through their entire bodies, not just watching onscreen or listening in class, but rather fully embodying and living in, with, and between.

Multiple Brains

When I work with children and parents, I introduce them to our multiple brains: head, heart, and gut (Soosalu, Henwood, & Deo, 2019). I may explore with the family biological factors such as identifying the chemicals, dopamine/serotonin in the gut as well as within the brain that drive our feelings of pleasure and desire for more. How to notice that mind-like experience in the belly when something doesn't feel right or when anticipating a big event and that swelling feeling felt in the heart when the child makes a meaningful connection and has a gleam in their eyes. Yet again, we see support for the imperative nature of body-based psychotherapeutic intervention for children, this time through the connection that exists between what is felt in the gut as well as within the brain (Porges, 2011). We activate and practice methods to support our vagus nerve and the connection through the belly, lungs, heart, throat, ears, nose, and brain. Dance/movement therapy methods activate the connected link from midline to the top of our head as we move our essential body parts, fostering true feelings and experiencing the world and relationships around us.

This snapshot of interpersonal neuroscience is the first layer of a system that builds to suggest how relationships with self and with others result in growth producing integration of the thinking/feeling/remembering aspects of one's brain; an integration that moves us toward a healthy mind and meaningful life.

(Delaney & Ferguson, 2014, p. 146)

Human Beingness

Finally, I share an analogy to other species: bears or bats. The bear has a heightened sense of smell, and the bat has a keen ability for sonar hearing: two intense, enormous sensory states felt in the body in what, I imagine, is unlike any other ability. But I can't imagine a bear or bat trying to rid themself of these abilities. Rather they embrace the senses as an aid in their survival. As humans, we make our existence so much harder than it has to be. If we don't honor our body/movement-based/feeling selves as aids in our survival, we are missing the experience of our amazing biology. We know that brain plasticity forms the framework for evolving, sifting, and consolidating; neurons fire and wire together, forming new pathways and chances for learning. The therapeutic relationship, in its use of movement, can be a conduit to achieving malleable, deeply intricate brain development and embodied existence.

Our society shines a benevolent light on individuals who rise from adversity to reach opportunity, but when we encounter adversity in our feelings and mental health, this concept gets lost. When we experience the feelings of others within ourselves, this is yet another chance to accept challenges as growth points and acknowledge the process that will unfold before us.

As mentioned throughout this book, in dance/movement therapy the body-based experience expressed through motion consistently represents a parallel process to the psychological and emotional states/needs of the individual. When we observe and then join in expressing true feelings in a safe environment within the clinical therapeutic space, we foster emotional healing and developmental growth. Therapeutic dance mirrors the dance of life, the interchange between bodies throughout history and within cultures, families, and diverse groups. Look around you: See how timing, whether the speed of natural growth or the slowness of evolution, underscores the closeness and depth of our everyday experiences; how weight, whether it's in the seemingly effortless gliding of birds or solid, secure mountains, exposes our true nature at every turn. Body knowledge is our birthright; let's give permission to children and expand our therapeutic tool kits by observing the child's needs, experiences, and expressed movements and enable emotional healing through the whole body. Identify the planes of movement in your interactions with clients, soothing from side to side, strength in upright posturing, and embracing in a forward motion.

Conclusion

You have read about the many *moving moments* dance/movement therapy sessions with children and parents. You received interventions and prompts to support a secure connection between parent and child, support for sibling communication, and between children and their community members, teachers, and doctors. These moments explored pain management, social isolation, anxiety, fear, sensory challenges, and even daily life skills such as sleep and transitions. You now have an embodied understanding of the transformative nature of utilizing a mind/body approach, play, and movement with children for therapeutic support. Take these concepts and stories and apply them to your daily interactions with children as a parent, educator, or professional. We all can have body knowledge, the ability to be aware of our personal preferences, the insight into our body's nonverbal communication patterns, and the creativity to support all meaningful learning. Let's all move together!

References

AACAP. (2024). *A declaration from the American academy of child and adolescent psychiatry, the American academy of pediatrics, and children's hospital association* (pp. 1–2). www.AACAP.org

Abram, D. (2011). *Becoming animal: An earthly cosmology*. Knopf Doubleday Publishing Group.

ADTA. (2020). *Frequently asked questions*. American Dance Therapy Association. Retrieved September 23, 2023. www.adta.org

Arain, M., Haque, M., Johal, L., Mathur, P., Nel, W., Rais, A., Sandhu, R., & Sharma, S. (2013). Maturation of the adolescent brain. *Neuropsychiatric Disease and Treatment*, 9, 449–461. https://doi.org/10.2147/NDT.S39776

CDC. (2023). *Disparities in Suicide*. Centers for Disease Control and Prevention, National Center for Injury Prevention and Control. www.cdc.org

Delahooke, M. (2019). *Beyond behaviors: Using brain science and compassion to understand and solve children's behavioral challenges*. PESI Publishing & Media.

Delaney, K. R., & Ferguson, J. (2014). Peplau and the brain: Why interpersonal neuroscience provides a useful language for the relationship process. *Journal of Nursing Education and Practice*, 4(8), 145.

Diamond, A. (2013). Executive functions. *Annual Review of Psychology*, 64, 135–168. https://doi.org/10.1146/annurev-psych-113011-143750

Gvion, Y., & Bar, N. (2014). Sliding doors: Some reflections on the parent–child–therapist triangle in parent work–child psychotherapy. *Journal of Child Psychotherapy*, 40(1), 58–72.

Healthy Children. (2023). Transitional objects, security blankets & beyond. In *Caring for your baby and young child: Birth to age 5* (7th Ed.). American Academy of Pediatrics. www.Healthychildren.org

Jeraka, T., Vidriha, A., & Žvelcb, G. (2018). The experience of attunement and misattunement in dance movement therapy workshops. *The Arts in Psychotherapy*, 60, 55–62.

Lambert, K., Eisch, A. J., Galea, L. A. M., Kempermann, G., & Merzenich, M. (2019). Optimizing brain performance: Identifying mechanisms of adaptive neurobiological plasticity. *Neuroscience and Biobehavioral Reviews*, 105, 60–71. https://doi.org/10.1016/j. neubiorev.2019.06.033

Leisman, G., Moustafa, A. A., & Shafir, T. (2016). Thinking, walking, talking: Integratory motor and cognitive brain function. *Frontiers in Public Health*, 4, 94. https://doi. org/10.3389/fpubh.2016.00094

Loman, S., & Sossin, M. K. (2016). The Kestenberg movement profile in dance/movement therapy: An introduction. In *The art and science of dance/movement therapy: Life is dance* (2nd Ed., Vol. 2, pp. 255–284). Routledge/Taylor & Francis Group.

Lopez, C., Falconer, C. J., & Mast, F. W. (2013). Being moved by the self and others: Influence of empathy on self-motion perception. *PLoS One*, 8(1), e48293.

Martin, D. J., Garske, J. P., & Davis, M. K. (2000). Relation of the therapeutic alliance with outcome and other variables: A meta-analytic review. *Journal of Consulting and Clinical Psychology*, 68(3), 438–450.

Novita, D., Suyono, S., & Yuanita, L. (2021). Dynamic equilibrium: The conception of a prospective chemistry teacher. *Advances in Engineering Research*, 209, 179–184.

Porges, S. W. (2011). *The polyvagal theory: Neurophysiological foundations of emotions, attachment, communication, and self-regulation* (Norton Series on Interpersonal Neurobiology). W. W. Norton & Company.

Sandhu, S., Arcidiacono, E., Aguglia, E., & Priebe, S. (2015). Reciprocity in therapeutic relationships: A conceptual review. *International Journal of Mental Health Nursing*, 24(6), 460–470.

Schwartz, J. M., Stapp, H. P., & Beauregard, M. (2005). Quantum physics in neuroscience and psychology: A neurophysical model of mind-brain interaction. *Philosophical Transactions of the Royal Society of London: Series B, Biological Sciences*, 360(1458), 1309–1327.

Siegel, D. J. (2022). *IntraConnected: MWe (Me + We) as the integration of self, identity, and belonging*. National Geographic Books.

Siegel, D. J., & Bryson, T. P. (2019). *The yes brain: How to cultivate courage, curiosity, and resilience in your child*. Random House Publishing Group.

Siegel, D. J., & Drullis, C. (2023). An interpersonal neurobiology perspective on the mind and mental health: Personal, public, and planetary well-being. *Annals of Psychiatry*, 22(5). https://doi.org/10.1186/s12991-023-00434-5

Soosalu, G., Henwood, S., & Deo, A. (2019). Head, heart, and gut in decision making: Development of a multiple brain preference questionaire. *Sage Open*, 9(1). https://doi. org/10.1177/2158244019837439

Vidick, T. (2023). What is entanglement and why is it important? *Caltech science exchange*. https://scienceexchange.caltech.edu/topics/quantum-science-explained/entanglement

Weber, R. (2022). *Movement therapy as an alternative to talk therapy*. Newsroom. University of Auckland.

About the Author and Co-Contributor

Dr. Lori Baudino, BC-DMT
Licensed Clinical Psychologist 22011

Dr. Lori Baudino has been a practicing clinician for over twenty years. She received her doctorate in clinical psychology and master's in creative arts therapy – dance/movement therapy, the therapeutic use of movement to further the emotional, cognitive, physical, and social integration of the individual.

As the National Clinical Spokesperson for The Andréa Rizzo Foundation, and with their funding, Dr. Baudino brought the first dance/movement therapy programs to top pediatric hospitals in Los Angeles, providing bedside therapy to children with cancer and special needs. Dr. Baudino offers professional development, advisory, and supervision within the field of mental health to support the integration of embodied practices for working with children.

Dr. Baudino, a distinguished expert in media news outlets supporting children, is a sought-after speaker at retreats, conferences, and workshops, and she is a dedicated member of the Garrison Fellowship program (Cohort II) for contemplative leaders, where she passionately focuses on global initiatives to bridge the gap in mental health care.

In her private practice, she works with children and their families to support the developing child and the integral relationships between parent, child, and siblings. Understanding the premise that the body, mind, and spirit are interconnected, and that life is experienced through movement, Dr. Baudino's approach allows the child to put words into action, understand individual sensory and motor preferences, express emotional needs, and support overall integration and well-being.

Dr. Baudino is also a published author, leveraging her love of travel with her expertise in child behavior to create the informational book, *Super Flyers: A Parent Guidebook for Airplane Travel With Children*.

SPECIALIZATION (But Not Limited To)

- Child Development
- Asychonistic/2e/Gifted/Neurodivergent
- Medically Fragile and Chronic Illness
- Special Needs/Autism Spectrum Disorder
- ADHD, Anxiety, Depression, and Additional Learning/Behavioral Challenges
- Addiction, Trauma, Early Intervention/Parent Support
- New Parenting/Infant Attachment
- Travel Preparation and Success
- Dance/Movement Therapy for Adult Integrative Wellness/Retreats/ Health Care

Contact

Email: Therapy@drloribaudino.com
Website: www.drloribaudino.com

Social Channels

Twitter: @drloribaudino
Facebook: Dr Lori Baudino
Instagram: @drloribaudino
Instagram: @superflyerstravel
Instagram: @global_therapists
YouTube: Dr Lori Baudino

Affiliations

American Psychological Association (APA)
American Dance Therapy Association (ADTA)
American Dance Movement Board
The Andréa Rizzo Foundation

Co-Contributor

Rachael Singer, BC-DMT
Board Certified Dance/Movement Therapist-1372

Rachael Singer is a board-certified dance/movement therapist and a senior case manager at Positive Development, Inc. Rachael began her career as a preschool teacher in Reggio Emilia inspired preschools. She received a Bachelor of Arts in child development and a Master of Science in dance/

movement therapy. Rachael is certified in the Profectum DIR Model, Level 1 and Level 2, and she is currently completing her DIR Trainer Certificate.

Rachael's experience working with children and families spans more than a decade. In 2016, she founded her counseling practice, Rachael's Moving HeARTS, LLC, where she facilitated parent and child support through dance/movement therapy. Rachael also shares her experience across multiple educational platforms, such as national conferences; summits; college courses; staff training; and workshops for teachers, paraprofessionals, clinicians, and families.

She currently supervises in-home developmental paraprofessionals and case managers and provides developmental care to children and adolescents on the autism spectrum as part of a transdisciplinary team in New Jersey. She created and implemented Mindful Movement for Positive Development, an employee resource group that offers all employees a thirty-minute mindful movement session for self-care.

Rachael had the honor and pleasure of having Dr. Lori Baudino as her supervisor when working at Real Connections Institute, supporting neurodiverse children and families through a developmental and play-based approach. After becoming close friends and colleagues, Rachael and Dr. Lori began to collaborate and work together on *Moving Moments*.

Thank you, Dr. Lori, from the bottom of my heart, for including me on this journey with you and for inspiring me to continue to not only advocate for our field of dance/movement therapy, but for the whole child, the whole family, and for myself.

Contact

Email: movinghearts11@gmail.com
Website: www.positivedevelopment.com

Social Channels

Instagram: @rachaelsmovinghearts

Index